Bariatrics for the Endoscopist

Guest Editor

CHRISTOPHER C. THOMPSON, MD

GASTROINTESTINAL ENDOSCOPY CLINICS OF NORTH AMERICA

www.giendo.theclinics.com

Consulting Editor
CHARLES J. LIGHTDALE, MD

April 2011 • Volume 21 • Number 2

SAUNDERS an imprint of ELSEVIER, Inc.

W.B. SAUNDERS COMPANY
A Division of Elsevier Inc.

1600 John F. Kennedy Blvd. • Suite 1800 • Philadelphia, Pennsylvania 19103-2899

http://www.giendo.theclinics.com

**GASTROINTESTINAL ENDOSCOPY CLINICS OF NORTH AMERICA Volume 21, Number 2
April 2011 ISSN 1052-5157, ISBN-13: 978-1-4557-0453-8**

Editor: Kerry Holland
Developmental Editor: Donald Mumford

Gastrointestinal Endoscopy Clinics of North America (ISSN 1052-5157) is published quarterly by Elsevier Inc., 360 Park Avenue South, New York, NY 10010-1710. Months of issue are January, April, July, and October. Business and Editorial Offices: 1600 John F. Kennedy Blvd., Suite 1800, Philadelphia, PA, 19103-2899. Periodicals postage paid at New York, NY and additional mailing offices. Subscription prices are $295.00 per year for US individuals, $414.00 per year for US institutions, $156.00 per year for US students and residents, $325.00 per year for Canadian individuals, $505.00 per year for Canadian institutions, $412.00 per year for international individuals, $505.00 per year for international institutions, and $217.00 per year for Canadian and foreign students/residents. To receive student/resident rate, orders must be accompanied by name of affiliated institution, date of term, and the *signature* of program/residency coordinator on institution letterhead. Orders will be billed at individual rate until proof of status is received. Foreign air speed delivery is included in all *Clinics* subscription prices. All prices are subject to change without notice. **POSTMASTER:** Send address change to *Gastrointestinal Endoscopy Clinics of North America*, Elsevier Health Sciences Division, Subscription Customer Service, 3251 Riverport Lane, Maryland Heights, MO 63043. **Customer Service: 1-800-654-2452 (US). From outside the United States, call 1-314-447-8871. Fax: 1-314-447-8029. E-mail: JournalsCustomerService-usa@elsevier.com (for print support) or JournalsOnlineSupport-usa@elsevier.com (for online support)**.

Reprints. For copies of 100 or more, of articles in this publication, please contact the Commercial Reprints Department, Elsevier Inc., 360 Park Avenue South, New York, NY 10010-1710. Tel. (212) 633-3812; Fax: (212) 482-1935; E-mail: reprints@elsevier.com.

Gastrointestinal Endoscopy Clinics of North America is covered in *Excerpta Medica, MEDLINE/PubMed (Index Medicus), and MEDLINE/MEDLARS.*

Printed and bound by CPI Group (UK) Ltd, Croydon, CR0 4YY

Transferred to Digital Print 2011

Contributors

CONSULTING EDITOR

CHARLES J. LIGHTDALE, MD
Professor, Department of Medicine, Columbia University Medical Center, New York, New York

GUEST EDITOR

CHRISTOPHER C. THOMPSON, MD
Assistant Professor of Medicine, Harvard Medical School; Director of Therapeutic Endoscopy, Director of Developmental Endoscopy Lab, Division of Gastroenterology, Brigham and Women's Hospital, Boston, Massachusetts

AUTHORS

BARHAM K. ABU DAYYEH, MD
Gastrointestinal Unit, Department of Medicine, Massachusetts General Hospital; Harvard Medical School, Boston, Massachusetts

DAN E. AZAGURY, MD
Bariatric and Minimally Invasive Surgery Fellow, Department of Surgery, Brigham and Women's Hospital, Harvard Medical School, Boston, Massachusetts

TODD H. BARON, MD, FASGE
Professor of Medicine, Mayo GI Bleeding Team, Division of Gastroenterology and Hepatology, Mayo Clinic, Rochester, Minnesota

BIPAN CHAND, MD
Director of Surgical Endoscopy, Bariatric and Metabolic Institute; Program Director, General Surgery Residency, Cleveland Clinic Main Campus, Cleveland, Ohio

ROGER A. DE LA TORRE, MD
Chief of General Surgery, Department of General Surgery, University Hospital, University of Missouri, Columbia, Missouri

LINCOLN E.V.V. FERREIRA, MD, PhD
Department of Medicine, Digestive Endoscopy Unit, Hospital Universitario da Universidade Federal de Juiz de Fora, Juiz de Fora, Minas Gerais, Brazil

GREGORY G. GINSBERG, MD
Professor of Medicine; Director of Endoscopy, Department of Medicine, Hospital of the University of Pennsylvania, Philadelphia, Pennsylvania

DANIEL M. HERRON, MD
Professor, Department of Surgery; Chief, Section of Laparoscopic and Bariatric Surgery, Mount Sinai School of Medicine, New York, New York

LEE M. KAPLAN, MD, PhD
Gastrointestinal Unit, Department of Medicine, Massachusetts General Hospital; Department of Medicine, Harvard Medical School, Boston, Massachusetts

JEANETTE N. KEITH, MD
Associate Professor of Medicine, Section of Gastroenterology, University of Buffalo, State University of New York; Director of Bariatric Medicine for Kaleida Health at Buffalo General Hospital, Buffalo New York

MOUEN A. KHASHAB, MD
Division of Gastroenterology and Hepatology, Department of Medicine, The Johns Hopkins Medical Institutions, Johns Hopkins University, Baltimore, Maryland

DAVID B. LAUTZ, MD
Director of Bariatric Surgery, Department of Surgery, Brigham and Women's Hospital; Assistant Professor of Surgery, Harvard Medical School, Boston, Massachusetts

MICHAEL J. LEE, MD
Department of Surgery, Southwestern Center for Minimally Invasive Surgery, University of Texas Southwestern Medical Center, Dallas, Texas

BRENT W. MIEDEMA, MD
Professor of Surgery, Department of General Surgery, University Hospital, University of Missouri, Columbia, Missouri

MARIO P. MORALES, MD
SSM Weight-Loss Institute, DePaul Health Center, SSM Health Care, St Louis, Missouri

PATRICK I. OKOLO III, MD, MPH
Division of Gastroenterology and Hepatology, Department of Medicine, The Johns Hopkins Medical Institutions, Johns Hopkins University, Baltimore, Maryland

OCTAVIA PICKETT-BLAKELY, MD, MHS
Instructor of Medicine, University of Pennsylvania School of Medicine, Gastroenterology Division, Hospital of the University of Pennsylvania, Philadelphia, Pennsylvania

RAMIN ROOHIPOUR, MD
Fellow, Mount Sinai School of Medicine, New York, New York

MICHELE B. RYAN, MS
Senior Research Lab Manager, Developmental Endoscopy Laboratory, Division of Gastroenterology, Brigham and Women's Hospital, Boston, Massachusetts

MARVIN RYOU, MD
Advanced Endoscopy Fellow, Partners Combined Program, Division of Gastroenterology, Brigham and Women's Hospital; Gastrointestinal Unit, Massachusetts General Hospital, Harvard Medical School, Boston, Massachusetts

STEVEN D. SCHWAITZBERG, MD
Associate Professor, Department of Surgery, Harvard Medical School, Boston; Chief, Department of Surgery, Cambridge Health Alliance, Cambridge, Massachusetts

DANIEL J. SCOTT, MD, FACS
Associate Professor of Surgery, Frank H. Kidd Jr, MD, Distinguished Professorship in Surgery, Department of Surgery; Director, Southwestern Center for Minimally Invasive Surgery, University of Texas Southwestern Medical Center, Dallas, Texas

J. STEPHEN SCOTT, MD
Medical Director, SSM Weight-Loss Institute, DePaul Health Center, SSM Health Care, St Louis, Missouri

NABIL TARIQ, MD
Fellow, Flexible Endoscopy and Advanced Laparoscopy, Cleveland Clinic, Cleveland, Ohio

CHRISTOPHER C. THOMPSON, MD
Assistant Professor of Medicine, Harvard Medical School; Director of Therapeutic Endoscopy, Director of Developmental Endoscopy Lab, Division of Gastroenterology, Brigham and Women's Hospital, Boston, Massachusetts

JOHN J. VARGO, MD, MPH
Associate Professor of Medicine, Cleveland Clinic Lerner College of Medicine; Acting Chairman Head, Section of Therapeutic and Hepatobiliary Endoscopy, Department of Gastroenterology and Hepatology, Digestive Disease Institute, Cleveland Clinic, Cleveland, Ohio

LOUIS M. WONG KEE SONG, MD
Associate Professor of Medicine, Mayo GI Bleeding Team, Division of Gastroenterology and Hepatology, Mayo Clinic, Rochester, Minnesota

Contents

Foreword **xiii**

Charles J. Lightdale

Preface **xv**

Christopher C. Thompson

Obesity Overview: Epidemiology, Health and Financial Impact, and Guidelines for Qualification for Surgical Therapy **189**

Dan E. Azagury and David B. Lautz

The aim of this article is to describe the context in which this issue of *Gastrointestinal Endoscopy Clinics of North America* is established. The authors review the current worldwide dimensions and trends of the obesity epidemic; associated mortality and comorbid diseases including diabetes, cancer, cardiovascular disease and obstructive sleep apnea; the financial impact of obesity; and current national and international guidelines for referral and qualification for surgical treatment of obesity.

Medical Therapy for Obesity **203**

Barham K. Abu Dayyeh and Lee M. Kaplan

The large number of people with mild to moderate obesity contribute more to its overall public health burdens than the smaller number of people with severe obesity. High-risk, high-efficacy strategies and population strategies focusing on lifestyle and behavioral modifications have failed to address the population burden of disease. An individualized approach is likely to provide the most effective management of this disease for the largest number of patients. This review discusses advances in pharmacologic therapies for obesity with a focus on currently approved drugs and those in later stages of development.

Bariatric Surgical Anatomy and Mechanisms of Action **213**

Daniel M. Herron and Ramin Roohipour

Because bariatric surgery is becoming increasingly common, gastroenterologists need to be familiar with the surgical and endoscopic anatomy of the operations in use today. This review focuses on the 4 most commonly performed bariatric operations in the United States: Roux-en-Y gastric bypass, adjustable gastric band, sleeve gastrectomy, and biliopancreatic diversion with duodenal switch. The anatomy and mechanism of action of each procedure is discussed and illustrated. Emphasis is placed on the endoscopic anatomy, with review of the commonly encountered complications. Emerging techniques and devices are reviewed.

Presurgical Evaluation and Postoperative Care for the Bariatric Patient 229

Nabil Tariq and Bipan Chand

With the increasing number of bariatric surgeries being performed, multiple specialties encounter bariatric patients. This article gives an overview of the comprehensive evaluation and preoperative preparation of a bariatric patient. Medical, psychological, and behavioral evaluation is discussed. The role of routine preoperative endoscopy is controversial but can be very important and may alter the operation performed. Immediate postoperative care is also addressed. Undergoing bariatric surgery is a lifelong commitment, and frequent follow up with reinforcement and monitoring for nutritional deficiencies is extremely important.

Medical Management of Postsurgical Complications: The Bariatric Surgeon's Perspective 241

Michael J. Lee and Daniel J. Scott

Bariatric surgery remains the only effective method to initiate and sustain massive weight loss in morbidly obese patients. Along with the advent of minimal access surgery, its popularity has not only resulted in an exponential increase in number of cases but also a subsequent increase in number of complications. Although most postsurgical bariatric complications are managed surgically, it is imperative that all physicians be aware of the unique potential complications to effectively communicate and optimize the medical management in this emergent set of patients.

Sedation in the Bariatric Patient 257

John J. Vargo

Obesity is a significant health problem that has assumed epidemic proportions. A durable reduction in weight and improved morbidity and mortality have been realized with the introduction of various bariatric surgical procedures. It is unknown how safe the current practices of sedation for endoscopic procedures are in bariatric patients. Morbid obesity can result in pulmonary hypertension, obstructive sleep apnea, and restrictive lung disease. This article explores these issues and how they may impact the risk profile of current standards for endoscopic sedation.

Endoscopy Unit Considerations in the Care of Obese Patients 265

Gregory G. Ginsberg and Octavia Pickett-Blakely

The dramatic increase in obesity in the general population is accompanied by a concomitant increase in bariatric surgical programs. Gastrointestinal endoscopy has an important role in patient evaluation, postoperative management, and emerging endoscopic bariatric therapies. Endoscopy units must address special design and equipment needs of obese patients in short- and long-range planning. Obese people require more health care resources than nonobese people, with increased physical challenges for staff in administering that care. This article details endoscopy unit considerations pertaining to the bariatric patient, which may apply to pretreatment endoscopic evaluation, managing postoperative bariatric surgical complications, and emerging endoluminal bariatric therapies.

Endoscopic Management of Common Bariatric Surgical Complications 275

Jeanette N. Keith

The primary role of endoscopic intervention in the care of bariatric surgery patients is in the management of late bariatric surgical complications and non-operative revision of the surgical anatomy. In the future, indications for therapeutic endoscopy will involve the gastroenterologist in primary weight loss interventions as cutting edge technology is currently undergoing rigorous scientific evaluation. Endoscopists caring for these patients should become familiar with post-bariatric surgical anatomy, potential complications, common presenting symptoms, anticipated luminal/extra-luminal findings, and endoscopic management of common bariatric complications; this review addresses these issues. This review will discuss common presenting symptoms, luminal as well as extra-luminal findings and endoscopic management of common bariatric complications.

Management of Acute Postoperative Hemorrhage in the Bariatric Patient 287

Lincoln E.V.V. Ferreira, Louis M. Wong Kee Song, and Todd H. Baron

Bariatric surgery is one of the treatment options for achieving and preserving weight loss and managing medical complications related to obesity. After bariatric surgery, early or late adverse events, such as intraluminal or extraluminal gastrointestinal hemorrhage, can occur. Early gastrointestinal bleeding is more often a complication associated with Roux-en-Y gastric bypass surgery than other bariatric procedures and usually arises from the gastrojejunal anastomosis. Early postoperative bleeding may be potentially life threatening, although death after postbariatric surgery as a consequence of acute bleeding is uncommon. Although early postoperative intraluminal bleeding can usually be managed conservatively, endoscopic therapy may be required.

Management of Postsurgical Leaks in the Bariatric Patient 295

Mario P. Morales, Brent W. Miedema, J. Stephen Scott, and Roger A. de la Torre

Postsurgical leaks after bariatric procedures are a significant cause of morbidity and mortality. They usually arise from anastomotic and staple line failures that are attributed to surgical technique, ischemia, and patient comorbid conditions. Timely diagnosis from subtle clinical clues is the key to appropriate management. Traditional treatment consists of adequate control of the intra-abdominal infection via surgical or percutaneous drainage maneuvers, antibiotics, and nutrition support via parenteral or feeding tube routes. Recently, endoscopically placed covered esophageal stents have been used to exclude the leak site, allowing oral nutrition and speeding healing.

Accessing the Pancreatobiliary Limb and ERCP in the Bariatric Patient 305

Mouen A. Khashab and Patrick I. Okolo III

The Roux-en-Y gastric bypass (RYGB) accounts for more than 60% of bariatric procedures performed in the United States today. The RYGB anatomy poses particular challenges to interventional endoscopists who intend to access the papilla. Deep enteroscopy-assisted endoscopic

FORTHCOMING ISSUES

July 2011

Stents

Todd Baron, MD, *Guest Editor*

October 2011

Upper Gastrointestinal Bleeding

Roy K.H. Wong, MD, *Guest Editor*

January 2012

Health Care Reform and Gastroenterology: 2012

John I. Allen, MD, MBA, AGAF and Mark DeLegge, MD, *Guest Editors*

RECENT ISSUES

January 2011

Advances in the Diagnosis and Management of Barrett's Esophagus

Irving Waxman, MD, FASGE, *Guest Editor*

October 2010

Quality Colonoscopy

John I. Allen, MD, MBA, AGAF, *Guest Editor*

July 2010

Non-Polypoid (Flat and Depressed) Colorectal Neoplasms

Roy Soetikno, MD and Tonya Kaltenbach, MD, *Guest Editors*

RELATED INTEREST

Gastroenterology Clinics of North America, March 2010 (Vol. 39, No. 1)
Gastroenterologic Issues in the Obese Patient
David A. Johnson, MD, *Guest Editor*

Foreword

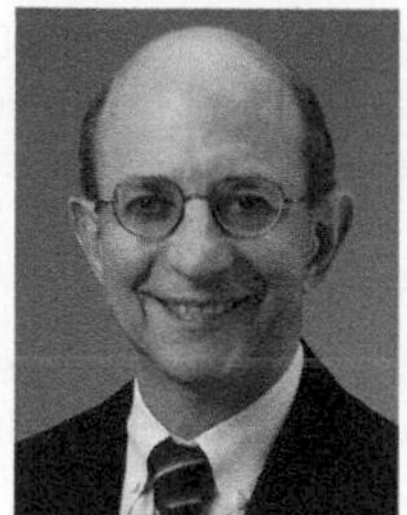

Charles J. Lightdale, MD
Consulting Editor

Evident from any casual observation in an airport, theme park, or stadium, obesity has emerged as the major public health menace of our time. Clearly linked to diabetes, cardiovascular disease, liver disease, and many cancers, obesity has become widely prevalent in our society in children and adults. While national attention has focused on a healthier food supply, diet control, and regular exercise for prevention of obesity, these measures often are insufficient for the already obese patient. Pharmacologic treatments have also been disappointing and sometimes dangerous. Bariatric surgery, which at first seemed a drastic approach, has now become commonplace and in wide demand. The surgical procedures alter upper GI anatomy to variably restrict food intake or cause malabsorption.

The role of the gastroenterologist has been mainly to understand the bariatric operations, recognize their long-term risks and side effects in ongoing management, and also to use flexible endoscopes to help reverse acute or chronic surgical complications. A new potential is the development of per-oral endoscopic therapies to reverse obesity. While past attempts have been fraught with only short-term efficacy and significant complications, novel approaches have great promise in this area. There is much to be learned and tested. New understanding of the neurologic and endocrine controls of appetite and satiety are also emerging from basic research that has the potential to be helpful in managing obesity. Gastroenterologists are going to have a central role in these efforts as well.

I was extremely pleased to have Dr Christopher Thompson as guest editor for this issue of the *Gastrointestinal Endoscopy Clinics of North America* devoted to the subject of obesity. Dr Thompson, of Brigham and Women's Hospital and Harvard Medical School, Boston, has been among the foremost advocates for gastrointestinal endoscopy's role in the management of obesity. In this state-of-the-art volume, he enlists a remarkable group of expert specialists to completely review the field. The

Gastrointest Endoscopy Clin N Am 21 (2011) xiii–xiv
doi:10.1016/j.giec.2011.03.001

need for endoscopic progress in this area is tremendous; the moment to rise to the challenge is now, and the key to progress is written here.

Charles J. Lightdale, MD
Department of Medicine
Columbia University Medical Center
161 Fort Washington Avenue, Room 812
New York, NY 10032, USA

E-mail address:
CJL18@columbia.edu

Preface

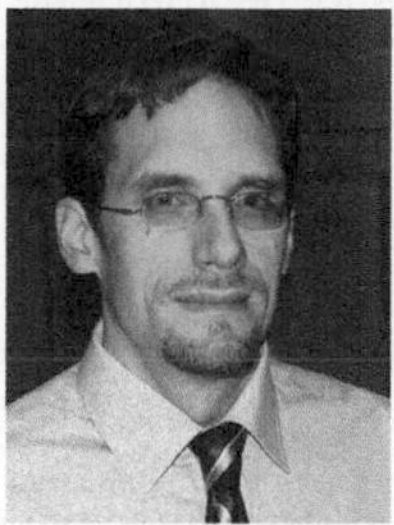

Christopher C. Thompson, MD
Guest Editor

In the United States approximately one in five individuals over 18 years of age is obese, and it is clear that this very real epidemic is rapidly becoming global in scope. Dietary programs, behavioral modification, and medical therapies have thus far provided inadequate long-term results. Bariatric surgery, however, does offer a means of durable weight loss for many patients with morbid obesity, and it is estimated that over 200,000 procedures are performed in the United States annually.

There are many types of weight loss surgery, and each specific procedure may have significant technical variations. These different surgeries and their procedural variants may in turn be associated with unique gastrointestinal complications. For example, circular staplers are more likely to lead to anastomotic strictures than linear staplers, and a longer Roux limb may make ERCP impossible with standard equipment. The endoscopist must understand these surgical procedures and their potential complications to provide an adequate standard of care for this emerging patient population. Additionally, it is critical to be familiar with local surgical techniques and to review surgical reports prior to scheduling endoscopy. This will lead to more effective procedures with more accurate choice of sedation and procedural setting, and will limit unnecessary procedures.

Furthermore, as endoscopic technologies have improved, the gastroenterologist has become increasingly effective in managing many of these complications. This includes basic methods for ulcer and stricture management, and more advanced techniques, such as the use of covered stents to treat postsurgical leaks and endoscopic suturing for the management of weight regain. Nevertheless, even what appears to be the most basic and familiar complication to the gastroenterologist has important differences in the bariatric patient. For example, in the management of marginal ulceration, biopsies of the gastric pouch and breath tests may not be adequate to exclude *Helicobacter pylori*, and foreign material may need to be removed for ulcer healing to occur. Similarly, 'over dilation' of anastomotic stenosis may lead to undesirable weight regain, a complication not encountered in other populations. Some techniques, such as those applied to treat postsurgical leaks and weight regain, may be more aggressive than those seen in traditional endoscopic practice; however, they are considerably less invasive than surgical alternatives and should be considered when relevant.

Gastrointest Endoscopy Clin N Am 21 (2011) xv–xvi
doi:10.1016/j.giec.2011.02.014
giendo.theclinics.com
1052-5157/11/$ – see front matter

Several novel devices are also now being investigated for the endoscopic treatment of obesity. These include but are not limited to balloons, gastric restriction devices, staplers, suturing platforms, implantable sleeves, and neuromodulatory devices. The reduced risk profile and unique mechanisms of action of these emerging technologies may provide new points of intervention for obese patients. Potential procedure categories include: Primary Obesity Procedures that may provide durable weight loss similar to conventional bariatric surgeries; Early Intervention Procedures to treat obesity that is not yet severe enough to meet criteria for traditional surgery; Bridge Procedures that induce short-term weight loss to reduce operative risk associated with morbid obesity; Metabolic Procedures that focus on obesity-related comorbid disease; and Revision Procedures that repair failed gastric bypass. The gastroenterologist has the endoscopic skill and technical ability necessary to perform these procedures; however, various cognitive elements regarding obesity management and postoperative care must be better understood to safely manage these patients.

Current management strategies are not effectively addressing the worsening obesity epidemic and it is now evident that a full spectrum of multidisciplinary care is needed. The best approach will involve noninvasive methods (diet, exercise, and education), medications, minimally invasive endoscopic techniques, and traditional surgery. The gastroenterologist can participate at many points along this spectrum and would likely benefit from improved integration into bariatric centers of excellence.

This issue of *Gastrointestinal Endoscopy Clinics of North America* is the work of a multidisciplinary group of experts and thought leaders and is intended to serve as a primer on the management of obese and bariatric patients. Epidemiology, pharmacological and surgical treatment of obesity, surgical anatomy, and postoperative complications are covered in detail. Additionally, emerging endoluminal weight loss procedures, regulatory issues, and economic concerns are examined.

Christopher C. Thompson, MD
Division of Gastroenterology
Brigham and Women's Hospital
Harvard Medical School
75 Francis Street
Boston, MA 02115, USA

E-mail address:
cthompson@hms.harvard.edu

Obesity Overview: Epidemiology, Health and Financial Impact, and Guidelines for Qualification for Surgical Therapy

Dan E. Azagury, MD*, David B. Lautz, MD

KEYWORDS

• Obesity • Body mass index • Disease risk quantification
• International guidelines • Bariatric surgery • Diabetes

The aim of this article is to describe the context in which this issue of *Gastrointestinal Endoscopy Clinics of North America* is established. The authors review the dimensions of the obesity epidemic, associated comorbid diseases, the impact of obesity, as well as current national and international guidelines for referral and qualification for surgical treatment of obesity.

DEFINITIONS

Many classifications have been used to measure and define obesity, and specifically to quantify the relationship between obesity and its impact on overall health and on the incidence of comorbidities and mortality.

The measurements used include waist circumference, total body fat, percent body fat, body mass index (BMI), and skin fold thickness. No single parameter has yet been able to adequately correlate obesity and its related comorbidities and to provide the optimal screening tool.[1] However, waist circumference (reflecting central obesity) has been described as potentially carrying the strongest association with cardiovascular disease risk factors when compared with other measures of adiposity.[2] Consequently, a threshold of 40 in (101.5 cm) in males and 35 in (89 cm) in females has been

No financial support.
No financial disclosures.
Department of Surgery, Brigham and Women's Hospital, Harvard Medical School, 75 Francis Street, Boston, MA 02115, USA
* Corresponding author.
E-mail address: dazagury@partners.org

Gastrointest Endoscopy Clin N Am 21 (2011) 189–201
doi:10.1016/j.giec.2011.02.001
giendo.theclinics.com
1052-5157/11/$ – see front matter

set for an increased risk of cardiovascular disease and other comorbidities. This threshold puts most patients with a BMI greater than 35 in an increased risk category, without further differentiation. This delineation is therefore currently more limited to the "leanest" of the obese patients, and its discriminating superiority over BMI is not clearly established.[3]

BMI remains the most widely used classification of obesity. It has been demonstrated to be a strong predictor of overall mortality[4] as well as to be directly associated with the presence of comorbidities.[5] Although BMI does not distinguish fat and lean body mass, it carries the advantage of being widely used, intuitive, and totally reproducible without operator-dependent or technique-dependent variations (such as skin fold thickness).[6] BMI also integrates undernutrition in the same measurement scale, with a good association with increased mortality in this population.[7] BMI is therefore the most commonly used screening tool in quantifying obesity and is used in most international guidelines.

The question of weight standards also remains imperfectly defined. In the past, the ideal weight range for an individual was determined according to standard tables published by insurance companies. These tables were based on the average weight and height of their customers, and a 20% margin was accepted above and below the average. The most famous of these tables were the Metropolitan Life Insurance Company data published in 1959 and 1983.[8,9] However, these tables were subject to a selection bias and included the notion of body frame size, making their use somewhat subjective. The subsequent adoption of BMI as a weight measurement tool has allowed organizations and experts to define an objective measurement tool as well as a standardized definition of normal weight range.

BMI is calculated by dividing weight in kilograms by the height in meters squared. Normal weight has a BMI ranging from 18.5 to 24.9 kg/m^2. A BMI under 18.5 is considered underweight while a BMI of 25 to 29.9 is defined as overweight. An individual is obese when their BMI is 30. There are 3 grades of obesity: grade 1 (BMI ranging from 30 to 34.9), grade 2 (BMI ranging from 35.0 to 39.9), and grade 3 (BMI $\geq$40) (**Table 1**).[10,11]

EPIDEMIOLOGY

For the past 20 years, scientific literature referring to the management of obesity typically included an introductory statement resembling the following: "obesity is becoming a health issue of epidemic proportions." However, this is no longer the

Table 1
Weight range classification

	Body Mass Index (kg/m^2)
Underweight	<18.5
Normal weight range	18.5–24.9
Overweight	>25
Pre-obesity	25–29.9
Obesity	>30
Grade 1 obesity	30–34.9
Grade 2 obesity	35–39.9
Grade 3 (morbid) obesity	>40

case. Obesity is no longer a developing health issue; it is a well-established pandemic that affected countries have not been able to tackle.

The past 2 to 3 decades have witnessed the development of a new field in surgery (bariatric surgery) directed at treating the most severe cases of obesity (BMI >35 or 40). This progress has included the creation of specialized centers, surgical fellowships, and scientific peer-reviewed journals devoted to the field.

However, the vast majority of patients do not qualify for such extreme surgical methods, and national or international attempts to deal with this disease have had little effect. As an illustration, 10 years ago the United States Department of Health and Human Services launched Healthy People 2010, a nationwide health promotion and disease prevention agenda.[12] The objectives of this project included addressing the issue of obesity and were developed with the Food and Drug Administration (FDA) and the National Institutes of Health (NIH). The aim was to promote health and reduce chronic disease associated with diet and weight in the United States, and included the following objectives to be achieved between 1999 and 2010:

1. Increase the proportion of adults who are at a healthy weight (BMI between 18.5 and 25) from 42% to 60%
2. Reduce the proportion of adults who are obese from 23% (data source: National Health and Nutrition Examination Survey [NHANES], Centers for Disease Control and Prevention [CDC], National Center for Health Statistics [NCHS]) to 15%
3. Reduce the proportion of children and adolescents who are overweight or obese from 11% (data source: NHANES, CDC, NCHS) to 5%.

At the same time (2001) the United States Surgeon General launched an "effort to develop an action plan to combat overweight/obesity."[13]

Ten years after this nationwide effort, and as the 2020 version of this agenda is under way, none of these objectives have been achieved. Furthermore, the latest data from the same source state that the increase in obesity prevalence is continuing at the same rate, and shows the following numbers for each objective for 2007 to 2008:

1. The proportion of adults who are at a healthy weight (BMI between 18.5 and 25) has *decreased* from 42% to 32% (goal was 60%)[14]
2. The proportion of adults who are obese has *increased* from 23% (data source: NHANES, CDC, NCHS) to 33.8% (goal was 15%)[14]
3. The proportion of overweight or obese children and adolescents has *increased* from 11% (data source: NHANES, CDC, NCHS) to 16.9% (goal was 5%).[15]

As one of the nations most heavily affected by obesity, these statistics for the United States demonstrate not only the magnitude of this disease but also the daunting task awaiting those who try to reverse the current trend.

International Data

Like the United States, much of the rest of the world is also widely affected and is facing similarly ineffective calls for action: the World Health Organization (WHO) report entitled *Obesity: Preventing and Managing the Global Epidemic* was published 10 years ago,[16] and worldwide prevalence of overweight and obesity have been continuously rising.[17] According to the WHO, 1.6 billion adults worldwide were overweight in 2005 and 400 million were obese, and estimations for 2015 are 2.3 billion and 700 million, respectively.

It is interesting that the United States is not the first country in terms of prevalence of obesity according to WHO data. The Pacific islands have a prevalence of obesity ranging from 40% in French Polynesia, to 78.5% in Nauru, followed by Saudi Arabia (35%), the United States (34%), countries of the Arabic peninsula (28%–33%), and New Zealand (26.5%).

Data comparison among countries remains limited, essentially because of differences in methodology of data collection, and most studies rely on telephonic surveys, gathering self-reported weights known to fault by underestimation.[18] For example, the Australian National Health Service measured data for 2007 to 2008 and reported 25% of adults as being obese, whereas self-reported BMI results from the survey showed "only" 21% of adults to be obese.[19]

Europe

Obesity was reported in 9.8% of Italian adults[20] in 2005, 12.9% of German adults in 2003,[21] and 16.9% of French adults in 2006.[22] In the United Kingdom, 24% of adults were classified as obese in 2006, compared with 15% in 1993.[23] The lowest incidence is found in Switzerland, with 8.1% in 2007.[24]

Asia

Many Asian countries have a low prevalence of obesity as defined by the BMI categories, yet high rates of obesity-related diseases.[25] In Japan, the prevalence of obesity was 3.1% in 2000,[26] whereas China reported a prevalence of obesity of 2.9% for 2002,[27] and only 0.46% of Vietnamese adults were obese in 2000.[28] However, a recent WHO expert panel concluded that Asians generally have a higher percentage of body fat than Caucasians of the same age, sex, and BMI. Also, the proportion of Asian people with risk factors for type 2 diabetes and cardiovascular disease is substantial even if below the existing WHO BMI cutoff point of 25. Indeed the WHO guidelines defining these cutoff points were based on data from Western countries. Therefore, a BMI greater than 23 is being considered as a potential threshold for increased weight-related health risk in these populations.[29,30]

Developing countries

Obesity is becoming a burden even in developing countries that are still struggling with malnutrition, with increasing prevalence particularly in urban areas. This phenomenon has been called the "double burden" of disease.[31] The WHO warns that the future burden of obesity and diabetes will significantly affect developing countries, and the projected numbers of new cases of diabetes run into the hundreds of millions within the next 2 decades.

MORTALITY AND COMORBID DISEASE

The WHO has analyzed the attributable number of deaths by risk factor around the world[32]: In 2004, obesity and overweight accounted for 11.4% of deaths in Europe and 9.5% of deaths in America (continent). In Europe, this was secondary only to high blood pressure (26.2%) and tobacco use (15.5%).

Little controversy remains regarding the relationship between obesity and increased incidence of comorbidities and mortality. The Framingham study in 1985 attributed a 3.9-times higher 30-year mortality rate to (nonsmoking) overweight men compared with nonobese men.[33] An analysis of this study demonstrated that a 40 year-old female nonsmoker loses 3.3 years and a male nonsmoker loses 3.1 years of life expectancy because of overweight. An obese female nonsmoker loses 7.1 years and males lose 5.8 years of life expectancy.[34]

In the recent past, some argument has remained as for the existence of a direct causative relationship between high BMI and increased mortality, and separating obesity from other closely related risk factors remains controversial. For example, a large cohort study of more than 20,000 patients has demonstrated that lean but unfit subjects had an overall mortality risk ratio double that of cardiorespiratorily fit obese patient (relative risk 2.06 vs 0.93) and comparable to unfit obese subjects (relative risk 1.92).[35] It now seems clear, however, that even if different risk factors intertwine and potentiate each other, and direct causality is not established, obesity is clearly related to a significant increase in overall mortality and specific comorbid diseases.

Some of the largest and most recent studies regarding BMI and mortality have not only demonstrated that obesity shortens life expectancy but also the linear relationship between the two. An analysis of 900,000 adults demonstrated that each 5 kg/m^2 higher BMI was on average associated with about 30% higher overall mortality[4]; and a study of nearly 1.5 million white adults reported that mortality increased both above a BMI of 25 and below a BMI of 20, with a hazard ratio of 2.51 in women with a BMI above 40 when compared with women with a BMI between 20 and 25.[36] In western Europe in 2000, 77% of subjects with a normal BMI are alive at age 70 years, but only 49% of subjects with a BMI between 40 and 50. Mortality from all causes was increased in obese patients, but cardiovascular death was the most important, followed by diabetes related death.

Comorbid Disease

Just as the relative role of each risk factor in increased mortality for overweight and obese patients is difficult to quantify, so is the causality of obesity in the existence of comorbid conditions. Yet the association of obesity with multiple comorbidities is clearly evident. A recent meta-analysis reviewed the associated risk of obesity and 18 comorbid conditions. The investigators found a positive association with 15 diseases, including type 2 diabetes; 6 cancer types: breast (postmenopausal), colorectal, endometrial, kidney, ovarian, and pancreatic; coronary artery disease; hypertension; pulmonary embolism; stroke; and asthma.[37] These results are detailed in **Table 2**.

Diabetes

Type 2 diabetes is one of the comorbid conditions with the closest demonstrated association with obesity. The incidence of type 2 diabetes worldwide has seen an increase that compares with that of obesity, and this combined epidemic trend has even been termed "diabesity."[38] In the United States, prevalence of diagnosed and undiagnosed diabetes among people aged 20 years or older in 2007 was 10.7%, that is, 23.5 million people, and type 2 diabetes accounts for 90% to 95% of these cases.[39] This figure represents an increase of more than 1 million cases per year since 2002 when the incidence was 8.7% (18 million). In addition to the parallel rate of prevalence increase between obesity and type 2 diabetes, the matching geographic prevalence of both diseases is explicit (**Figs. 1** and **2**).

In a meta-analysis, the relative risk increase of type 2 diabetes was 1.2 for each unit of BMI,[40] and the risk appears increased in women. Indeed, the Nurse's Study revealed that a woman with a BMI greater than 35 had an age-adjusted relative risk of type 2 diabetes of 93 when compared with a woman with a BMI of less than 22.[41] In comparison, the male health professionals study found a relative risk of diabetes of (only) 42 in men with a BMI greater than 35 when compared with subjects with a BMI of less than 23.[42]

Table 2
Relative comorbidity risks related to being overweight or obese

Comorbidity	Overweight		Obese	
	Male	Female	Male	Female
Type 2 diabetes[a]	2.40 (2.12–2.72)	3.92 (3.10–4.97)	6.74 (5.55–8.19)	12.41 (9.03–17.06)
Cancer				
Breast, postmenopausal	—	1.08 (1.03–1.14)	—	1.13 (1.05–1.22)
Colorectal	1.51 (1.37–1.67)	1.45 (1.30–1.62)	1.95 (1.59–2.39)	1.66 (1.52–1.81)
Endometrial	—	1.53 (1.45–1.61)	—	3.22 (2.91–3.56)
Esophageal	1.13 (1.02–1.26)	1.15 (0.97–1.36)	1.21 (0.97–1.52)	1.20 (0.95–1.53)
Kidney	1.40 (1.31–1.49)	1.82 (1.68–1.98)	1.82 (1.61–2.05)	2.64 (2.39–2.90)
Ovarian	—	1.18 (1.12–1.23)	—	1.28 (1.20–1.36)
Pancreatic	1.28 (0.94–1.75)	1.24 (0.98–1.56)	2.29 (1.65–3.19)	1.60 (1.17–2.20)
Prostate	1.14 (1.00–1.31)	—	1.05 (0.85–1.30)	—
Cardiovascular Diseases				
Hypertension[a]	1.28 (1.10–1.50)	1.65 (1.24–2.19)	1.84 (1.51–2.24)	2.42 (1.59–3.67)
Coronary artery disease[a]	1.29 (1.18–1.41)[b]	1.80 (1.64–1.98)	1.72 (1.51–1.96)[b]	3.10 (2.81–3.43)
Congestive heart failure[a]	1.31 (0.96–1.79)	1.27 (0.68–2.37)[b]	1.79 (1.24–2.59)	1.78 (1.07–2.95)[b]
Pulmonary embolism	1.91 (1.39–2.64)	1.91 (1.39–2.64)	3.51 (2.61–4.73)	3.51 (2.61–4.73)
Stroke[a]	1.23 (1.13–1.34)[b]	1.15 (1.00–1.32)[b]	1.51 (1.33–1.72)[b]	1.49 (1.27–1.74)[b]
Other				
Asthma	1.20 (1.08–1.33)[b]	1.25 (1.05–1.49)[b]	1.43 (1.14–1.79)[b]	1.78 (1.36–2.32)[b]
Gallbladder disease[a]	1.09 (0.87–1.37)[c]	1.44 (1.05–1.98)[c]	1.43 (1.04–1.96)[c]	2.32 (1.17–4.57)[c]
Osteoarthritis	2.76 (2.05–3.70)	1.80 (1.75–1.85)[b]	4.20 (2.76–6.41)	1.96 (1.88–2.04)[b]
Chronic back pain	1.59 (1.34–1.89)[b]	1.59 (1.34–1.89)[b]	2.81 (2.27–3.48)[b]	2.81 (2.27–3.48)[b]

Cancer: cases, not mortality and indicated by physician diagnosis of cancer. Coronary artery disease: indicated by myocardial infarction or angina. Osteoarthritis: indicated by joint replacement. Chronic back pain: indicated by early retirement due to back pain.

[a] Waist circumference measures were considered to be a better risk predictor than body mass index measures.

[b] The relative risks calculated from the ratios of proportions (RR-Ps) were used; otherwise, the incidence rate ratios (IRRs) were used.

[c] Both RR-Ps and IRRs were used.

Data from Guh D, Zhang W, Bansback N, et al. The incidence of comorbidities related to obesity and overweight: a systematic review and meta-analysis. BMC Public Health 2009;9:88.

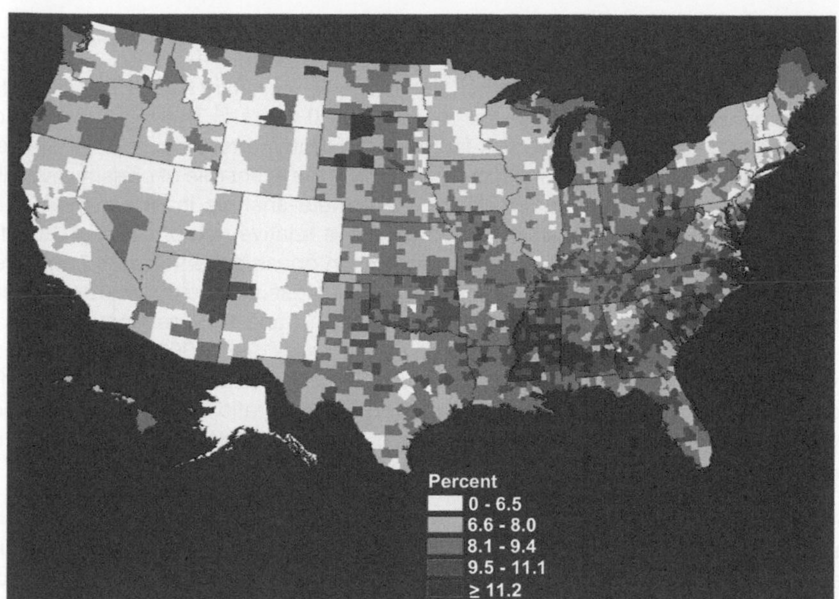

Fig. 1. Estimates of diagnosed diabetes for adults age 20 years and older: United States, 2004. (*Reproduced* with permission from CDC.)

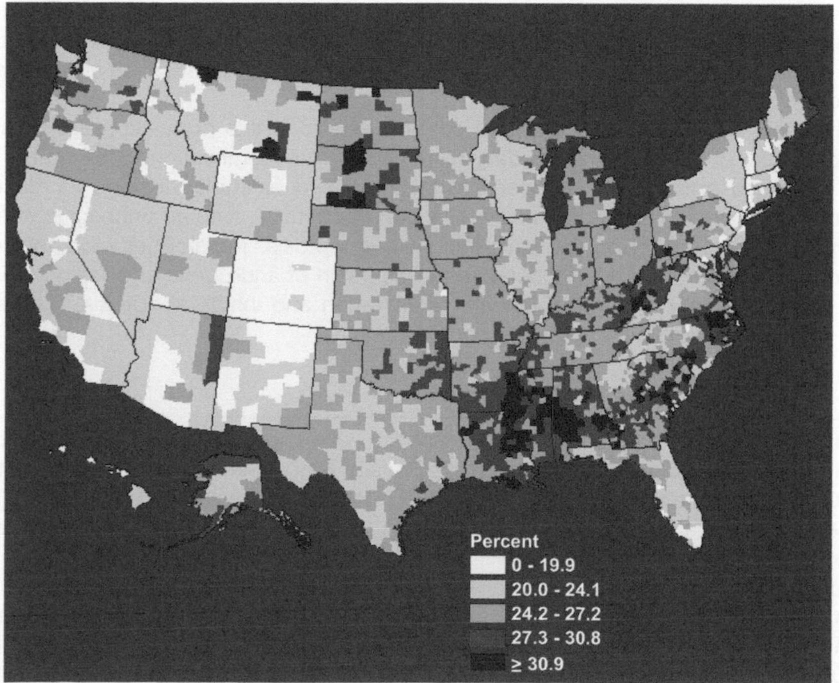

Fig. 2. Estimates of obesity among adults older than 20 years: United States, 2004. (*Reproduced* with permission from CDC.)

Cardiovascular Disease

Coronary heart disease

Obesity has been a known and declared risk factor for coronary heart disease (CHD) by the American Heart Association for more than 10 years.[43] The high association between obesity and other known risk factors of CHD (hypertension, hypercholesterolemia, and so forth) have made it difficult to quantify the exact role of obesity, even if it is a known independent risk factor. In a recent meta-analysis involving more than 300,000 patients, Bogers and colleagues[44] found a relative risk of CHD of 1.32 for patients with a BMI between 25 and 30, and 1.81 in obese patients when compared with nonobese patients. After adjusting for blood pressure and cholesterol levels, the relative risk was reduced but still significant at 1.17 and 1.49, respectively.

In addition, in a recent article reviewing NHANES data (1999–2004), the prevalence of hypertension increased from 18.1% for patients with normal weight to 52.3% for patients with a BMI greater than 40, with an adjusted odds ratio of 4.8. The prevalence of dyslipidemia in the same study increased from 8.9% to 19.0%, respectively, with an adjusted odds ratio of 2.0.[45]

Stroke

In a large meta-analysis including more than 2 million patients, Strazzullo and colleagues[46] found the relative risk was 1.64 for ischemic stroke and 1.24 for hemorrhagic stroke in obese patients as compared with subjects with a normal BMI.

Cancer

The increased incidence of cancer in obese patients has been well demonstrated for cancer of the colon, breast, endometrium, kidney, esophagus and gastric cardia, pancreas, gallbladder, and liver.[47] More specifically, a BMI greater than 30 carries a relative risk of colorectal cancer of 2 for men and 1.5 for women[48]; the relative risk of breast cancer is 1.5 for postmenopausal women[49] and 3.5 for endometrial cancer.[50]

The mechanisms behind increased carcinogenesis in this population are mostly hypothetical, but likely are secondary to the hormonal modifications attributable to the increased presence of adipose tissue. Proposed examples include increased circulating levels of insulin and insulin-like growth factor 1, with an unspecific effect promoting cellular proliferation and inhibiting apoptosis. Possibilities also include specific modifications such as increased conversion of androgens and testosterone into estrogens, which promote cellular proliferation and inhibit apoptosis in breast and endometrial cells.

Obstructive Sleep Apnea

Consequences of obstructive sleep apnea (OSA) range from motor vehicle accidents[51] to cardiovascular disease.[52] Obesity is the most important risk factor for OSA and is present in approximately 70% of patients with this disorder.[53] The underlying mechanisms are unclear, but probably include decreased pharyngeal airway size secondary to fat deposition, altered chest mechanics, and a genetic predisposition.[54]

In a recent prospective cohort study, weight management was shown to have a significant impact on the severity and occurrence of OSA: relative to stable weight, a 10% weight gain predicted an approximate 32% increase in the apneic episodes, a 10% weight loss predicted a 26% decrease, and a 10% increase in weight predicted a sixfold increase in the odds of developing moderate to severe OSA.[55]

FINANCIAL BURDEN OF DISEASE

According to the WHO, in 2004 overweight and obesity accounted for the loss of more than 35.8 million disability-adjusted life years (DALYs) worldwide.[32] The DALY extends the concept of potential years of life lost due to premature death to include equivalent years of "healthy" life lost by virtue of being in states of poor health or disability. The cost of obesity in the United States has been analyzed by Finkelstein and colleagues,[56] who estimated the total medical cost of obesity to be $147 billion in 2008, nearly doubling the estimation of 1998. This figure represented an annual spending of $1429 per person (42% higher than nonobese individuals). Nonmedical spending includes absenteeism and decreased income. The latter is difficult to quantify even if multiple studies have shown a negative relationship, especially in women.[57] Sick leave charges due to obesity-related absenteeism were estimated to cost $2.4 billion in 1998.[58]

QUALIFICATION FOR SURGERY AND GUIDELINES

If the burden of obesity is a complex health policy issue, treatment options for morbid obesity have been repeatedly disappointing. However, bariatric surgery has proven to be the first and most successful treatment for this population, leading to a rapid and exponential increase in the practice of this surgical specialty. In 2008, more than 220,000 bariatric surgical procedures were performed in North America.[59] National and professional guidelines have been edited to frame the indications for this surgery and its reimbursement.

Bariatric surgery is unique in that the patient is the initiator of treatment. Patients are able to decide if they wish to pursue such surgery, when they want surgery, and even the preferred type of procedure they wish to undergo. And even if the overall health benefits of weight reduction surgery are evident to the health care professional, the patient must have a strong autonomous will to pursue this route and initiate the process leading to surgery.

Important to this patient-initiated system is comprehensive public education. The available surgical options may also be limited to one procedure type by the surgeon and the multidisciplinary team. Although there are currently no formal guidelines regarding which patient should undergo which procedure, the preoperative workup is designed to determine to which procedure the patient is best suited. During this multidisciplinary workup the patient's medical history, including BMI, perioperative risk factors, metabolic variables, and comorbidities, are collected, all of which play a role in deciding the most appropriate procedure. Ultimately, however, the patient chooses a procedure with whose consequences they feel comfortable, based on their understanding of the risks and benefits of the available therapeutic options. The evaluation includes physical, psychiatric, and nutritional assessments, and ensures that the patient fulfills the current national criteria (eg, NIH) as a suitable bariatric surgery candidate. A secondary aim is to assist the candidate, often overwhelmed with information, to base his or her decision on correct and comprehensive information. Most importantly, the patient must be cognizant of the relative risks and benefits of the surgical procedure as compared with nonsurgical methods of weight loss. The patient's preparation therefore includes accurate and precise information regarding postsurgical care, and includes knowledge of short-term and long-term complications but also of short-term and long-term dietary restrictions, modifications, and supplementation.

Current national recommendations/policies for qualification of a patient for bariatric surgery are as follows.

NIH: BMI 40 or more, or BMI 35 or more and either of high-risk comorbid conditions such as life-threatening cardiopulmonary problems, severe diabetes mellitus, or obesity-induced physical problems interfering with lifestyle. The FDA is analyzing and may approve a request for use of one type of laparoscopic gastric band in patients with a BMI greater than 30.[60]

Most European countries require a BMI of 40 or greater and at least 2 weight-related comorbidities to qualify for bariatric surgery.

Other recommendations vary slightly depending on the country, and some additional requirements are specific to certain insurance companies. These recommendations/requirements often include a requirement that patients must have demonstrated failure of weight loss after 6 months of well conducted, followed-up nonsurgical treatment with dietary regimen, exercise, and behavioral support.

SUMMARY

Obesity carries an important toll on patient life expectancy and life-long risk of disease. Little is known about the underlying mechanisms of obesity or its associated comorbid illnesses, and effective treatment options are limited. Although surgical procedures have been proved to succeed in treating the most severe cases, the vast majority of patients in this pandemic remain confronted with the severe consequences of their obesity, with very few, if any, successful therapeutic options.

REFERENCES

1. Poirier P. Adiposity and cardiovascular disease: are we using the right definition of obesity? Eur Heart J 2007;28(17):2047–8.
2. Menke A, Muntner P, Wildman RP, et al. Measures of adiposity and cardiovascular disease risk factors. Obesity (Silver Spring) 2007;15(3):785–95.
3. Huxley R, Mendis S, Zheleznyakov E, et al. Body mass index, waist circumference and waist:hip ratio as predictors of cardiovascular risk–a review of the literature. Eur J Clin Nutr 2010;64(1):16–22.
4. Whitlock G, Lewington S, Sherliker P, et al. Body-mass index and cause-specific mortality in 900 000 adults: collaborative analyses of 57 prospective studies. Lancet 2009;373(9669):1083–96.
5. Qiao Q, Nyamdorj R. Is the association of type II diabetes with waist circumference or waist-to-hip ratio stronger than that with body mass index? Eur J Clin Nutr 2010;64(1):30–4.
6. Ulijaszek SJ, Kerr DA. Anthropometric measurement error and the assessment of nutritional status. Br J Nutr 1999;82(3):165–77.
7. Pednekar MS, Hakama M, Hebert JR, et al. Association of body mass index with all-cause and cause-specific mortality: findings from a prospective cohort study in Mumbai (Bombay), India. Int J Epidemiol 2008;37(3):524–35.
8. Metropolitan Life Insurance Company. New weight standards for men and women. Stat Bull Metropol Life Insur Co 1959;40:1–4.
9. Metropolitan Life Insurance Company MLI. Metropolitan height and weight tables. Stat Bull Metropol Life Insur Co 1983;64:2–9.
10. NIH. Health implications of obesity. NIH Consens Statement 1985;5(9):1–7.
11. NIH. Gastrointestinal surgery for severe obesity. NIH Consens Statement 1991; 9(1):1–20.
12. Office of Disease Prevention and Health Promotion. Healthy people 2010. US Department of Health and Human Services; 2000. Available at: http://www.healthypeople.gov/2010. Accessed March 9, 2011.

13. Office of the Surgeon General. Surgeon general launches effort to develop action plan to combat overweight obesity; 2001. Available at: http://www.surgeongeneral.gov/news/pressreleases/obesitypressrelease.htm. Accessed March 9, 2011.
14. Flegal KM, Carroll MD, Ogden CL, et al. Prevalence and trends in obesity among US adults, 1999–2008. JAMA 2010;303(3):235–41.
15. Ogden CL, Carroll MD, Curtin LR, et al. Prevalence of high body mass index in US children and adolescents, 2007–2008. JAMA 2010;303(3):242–9.
16. Obesity: preventing and managing the global epidemic. Report of a WHO consultation. World Health Organ Tech Rep Ser 2000;894:i–xii, 1–253.
17. WHO. WHO Fact sheet No 311: obesity and overweight. 2006. Available at: http://www.who.int/mediacentre/factsheets/fs311/en/. Accessed March 8, 2011.
18. Keith SW, Fontaine KR, Pajewski NM, et al. Use of self-reported height and weight biases the body mass index-mortality association. Int J Obes (Lond) 2010. [Epub ahead of print].
19. American Bureau of Statistics. National Health Survey: summary of results 2007–2008. Available at: http://www.abs.gov.au/ausstats/abs@.nsf/mf/4364.0/. Accessed March 9, 2011.
20. Istituto Nazionale di Statistica. Condizioni di salute, fattori di rischio e ricorso ai servizi sanitari [Health condition, risk factors and the use of health services]. Italy: Istituto Nazionale di Statistica; 2007. Available at: http://www.istat.it/salastampa/comunicati/non_calendario/20070302_00/testointegrale.pdf. Accessed March 9, 2011.
21. Rubner-Institut Bundesforschungsinstitut für Ernährung und Lebensmittel. Nationale Verzehrs Studie II—Ergebnisbericht Teil 1. Die bundesweite Befragung zur Ernährung von Jugendlichen und Erwachsenen. Karlsruhe (Germany): Max Rubner-Institut; 2008.
22. Institut de Veille Sanitaire. Etude nationale nutrition sante (ENNS, 2006)—Situation nutritionnelle en France en 2006 selon les indicateurs d'objectif et les reperes du programme national nutrition santé (PNNS) 2007. Available at: http://www.invs.sante.fr/surveillance/nutrition/enns.htm. Accessed March 9, 2011.
23. Statistics on obesity, physical activity and diet. England: NHS; 2008.
24. Office Fédéral De La Statistique. Enquête Suisse sur la santé (ESS). Neuchatel (Switzerland): OFS; 2007.
25. Khan NC, Khoi HH. Double burden of malnutrition: the Vietnamese perspective. Asia Pac J Clin Nutr 2008;17(Suppl 1):116–8.
26. Yoshiike N, Kaneda F, Takimoto H. Epidemiology of obesity and public health strategies for its control in Japan. Asia Pac J Clin Nutr 2002;11(Suppl 8):S727–31.
27. Ministry of Health, Ministry of Science and Technology, National Bureau of Statistics. The nutrition and health status of the Chinese people 2002. Beijing (China): International Life Science Institute(ILSI); 2004.
28. National Institute of Nutrition. General Nutrition Study. Hanoi (Vietnam): Medical Publishing House; 2003.
29. Choo V. WHO reassesses appropriate body-mass index for Asian populations. Lancet 2002;360(9328):235.
30. WHO Expert Consultation. Appropriate body-mass index for Asian populations and its implications for policy and intervention strategies. Lancet 2004; 363(9403):157–63.
31. Prentice AM. The emerging epidemic of obesity in developing countries. Int J Epidemiol 2006;35(1):93–9.
32. Risk factors estimates. 2004. Available at: http://www.who.int/healthinfo/global_burden_disease/risk_factors/en/index.html. Accessed December 27, 2010.

33. Garrison RJ, Castelli WP. Weight and thirty-year mortality of men in the Framingham Study. Ann Intern Med 1985;103(6 Pt 2):1006–9.
34. Peeters A, Barendregt JJ, Willekens F, et al. Obesity in adulthood and its consequences for life expectancy: a life-table analysis. Ann Intern Med 2003;138(1): 24–32.
35. Lee CD, Blair SN, Jackson AS. Cardiorespiratory fitness, body composition, and all-cause and cardiovascular disease mortality in men. Am J Clin Nutr 1999;69(3): 373–80.
36. Berrington de Gonzalez A, Hartge P, Cerhan JR, et al. Body-mass index and mortality among 1.46 million white adults. N Engl J Med 2010;363(23):2211–9.
37. Guh DP, Zhang W, Bansback N, et al. The incidence of co-morbidities related to obesity and overweight: a systematic review and meta-analysis. BMC Public Health 2009;9:88.
38. Zimmet P, Alberti KG, Shaw J. Global and societal implications of the diabetes epidemic. Nature 2001;414(6865):782–7.
39. Centers for Disease Control and Prevention. National diabetes fact sheet: general information and national estimates on diabetes in the United States, 2007. Atlanta (GA): U.S. Department of Health and Human Services; 2008.
40. Hartemink N, Boshuizen HC, Nagelkerke NJ, et al. Combining risk estimates from observational studies with different exposure cutpoints: a meta-analysis on body mass index and diabetes type 2. Am J Epidemiol 2006;163(11):1042–52.
41. Colditz GA, Willett WC, Rotnitzky A, et al. Weight gain as a risk factor for clinical diabetes mellitus in women. Ann Intern Med 1995;122(7):481–6.
42. Chan JM, Rimm EB, Colditz GA, et al. Obesity, fat distribution, and weight gain as risk factors for clinical diabetes in men. Diabetes Care 1994;17(9):961–9.
43. Eckel RH, Krauss RM. American Heart Association call to action: obesity as a major risk factor for coronary heart disease. AHA Nutrition Committee. Circulation 1998;97(21):2099–100.
44. Bogers RP, Bemelmans WJ, Hoogenveen RT, et al. Association of overweight with increased risk of coronary heart disease partly independent of blood pressure and cholesterol levels: a meta-analysis of 21 cohort studies including more than 300 000 persons. Arch Intern Med 2007;167(16):1720–8.
45. Nguyen NT, Magno CP, Lane KT, et al. Association of hypertension, diabetes, dyslipidemia, and metabolic syndrome with obesity: findings from the National Health and Nutrition Examination Survey, 1999 to 2004. J Am Coll Surg 2008; 207(6):928–34.
46. Strazzullo P, D'Elia L, Cairella G, et al. Excess body weight and incidence of stroke: meta-analysis of prospective studies with 2 million participants. Stroke 2010;41(5):e418–26.
47. Calle EE, Kaaks R. Overweight, obesity and cancer: epidemiological evidence and proposed mechanisms. Nat Rev Cancer 2004;4(8):579–91.
48. International Agency for Research on Cancer. Handbooks of cancer prevention. Weight Control and Physical Activity. Lyon (France): The International Agency for Research on Cancer (IARC); 2002.
49. Galanis DJ, Kolonel LN, Lee J, et al. Anthropometric predictors of breast cancer incidence and survival in a multi-ethnic cohort of female residents of Hawaii, United States. Cancer Causes Control 1998;9(2):217–24.
50. Ballard-Barbash R, Swanson CA. Body weight: estimation of risk for breast and endometrial cancers. Am J Clin Nutr 1996;63(Suppl 3):437S–41S.

51. Tregear S, Reston J, Schoelles K, et al. Continuous positive airway pressure reduces risk of motor vehicle crash among drivers with obstructive sleep apnea: systematic review and meta-analysis. Sleep 2010;33(10):1373–80.
52. Ramar K, Caples SM. Cardiovascular consequences of obese and nonobese obstructive sleep apnea. Med Clin North Am 2010;94(3):465–78.
53. Malhotra A, White DP. Obstructive sleep apnoea. Lancet 2002;360(9328):237–45.
54. Romero-Corral A, Caples SM, Lopez-Jimenez F, et al. Interactions between obesity and obstructive sleep apnea: implications for treatment. Chest 2010; 137(3):711–9.
55. Peppard PE, Young T, Palta M, et al. Longitudinal study of moderate weight change and sleep-disordered breathing. JAMA 2000;284(23):3015–21.
56. Finkelstein EA, Trogdon JG, Cohen JW, et al. Annual medical spending attributable to obesity: payer-and service-specific estimates. Health Aff (Millwood) 2009;28(5):w822–31.
57. Finkelstein EA, Ruhm CJ, Kosa KM. Economic causes and consequences of obesity. Annu Rev Public Health 2005;26:239–57.
58. Thompson D, Edelsberg J, Kinsey KL, et al. Estimated economic costs of obesity to U.S. business. Am J Health Promot 1998;13(2):120–7.
59. Buchwald H, Oien DM. Metabolic/bariatric surgery worldwide 2008. Obes Surg 2009;19(12):1605–11.
60. FDA. FDA executive summary memorandum; 2010.

Medical Therapy for Obesity

Barham K. Abu Dayyeh, MD[a,b], Lee M. Kaplan, MD, PhD[a,b,*]

KEYWORDS

- Obesity • Diet • Lifestyle modification • Medications
- Pharmacotherapy

Obesity and its associated conditions, including type 2 diabetes and cardiovascular disease, have reached epidemic proportions. This development is particularly evident in the developed world, where the consequences include substantially increased morbidity, mortality, and cost to the health care system.[1] In a recent meta-analysis of 89 prospective studies, obesity was significantly associated with at least 18 comorbid conditions that can be generally categorized into the following groups: metabolic disorders (including type 2 diabetes mellitus), cardiovascular disease, pulmonary, gastrointestinal (GI) and musculoskeletal complications, and cancer.[2] Studies from the National Health and Nutrition Examination Survey show that approximately one-third of the adult US population has obesity, that nearly 40% of these individuals have metabolic syndrome, and 1 in 7 have type 2 diabetes.[3,4]

The risks associated with obesity lie on a continuum. According to Geoffrey Rose's prevention paradox,[5] the large number of people with mild to moderate obesity contribute more to its associated public health burden than the small number of people with more severe forms of this disorder. Nonetheless, severe obesity is more commonly associated with comorbid disorders, and the burden of disease for each individual with severe obesity is disproportionately greater. Specialized treatments for this severely affected population, including GI weight loss surgery (GIWLS), are associated with too much risk to be applied to the broader population with obesity. The challenge in addressing obesity therefore lies in dealing with both sick individuals and a sick population.

Although population-based strategies, focusing on lifestyle and behavioral modifications, provide the greatest public health benefit overall, their long-term efficacy

---

Financial disclosures: BKAD – Nothing to disclose; LMK – Research support from Johnson & Johnson; scientific advisor to Merck Research Laboratories, Johnson & Johnson, GI Dynamics, Rhythm Pharmaceuticals, Gelesis, and Medtronic.

[a] Gastrointestinal Unit, Department of Medicine, Massachusetts General Hospital, 55 Fruit Street, Boston, MA 02114, USA

[b] Department of Medicine, Harvard Medical School, 25 Shattuck Street, Boston, MA, USA

* Corresponding author. Gastrointestinal Unit, Department of Medicine, Massachusetts General Hospital, 55 Fruit Street, Boston, MA 02114.

E-mail address: LMKaplan@partners.org

Gastrointest Endoscopy Clin N Am 21 (2011) 203–212
doi:10.1016/j.giec.2011.02.006 giendo.theclinics.com
1052-5157/11/$ – see front matter

has been limited.[6] The basis for this limitation is much debated, but biologic factors and the physiologic response to a changed environmental milieu play a role.[7,8]

A graded approach, akin to the management of hypertension, type 2 diabetes, and other chronic diseases seems likely to provide the greatest opportunity for clinical success. This approach, enabled by the development of a spectrum of new therapies, likely enables clinicians to make meaningful progress in the treatment of this epidemic. Potential contributors to this multifaceted approach include changes in diet composition, increased physical activity, and the sequential addition of nutritional, pharmacologic, endoscopic, and minimally invasive surgical therapies as needed.

Recent advances in our understanding of the mechanisms by which Roux-en-Y gastric bypass and other types of GIWLS induce profound, long-term weight loss and improvements in diabetes and other metabolic sequelae of obesity, combined with emerging endoscopic technologies, have opened the door to using endoscopic approaches to reproduce many of the benefits of bariatric surgery and thereby contribute to the effective treatment of obesity and its associated disorders. Early results are encouraging and suggest that endoscopy-based therapies may provide the next major treatment advance in this area. Progress in the development of new pharmacologic agents for obesity has been more limited. Despite extensive research and development efforts, few new pharmacologic agents have made their way into clinical practice for the primary management of obesity during the past 40 years. Of the currently available medications approved for the treatment of obesity, orlistat is the one most recently approved by the US Food and Drug Administration (FDA) for this indication, and it was approved in 1999.[9] The absence of newer agents reflects the modest effectiveness of recently developed weight loss medications, combined with safety profiles that have been considered unacceptable by FDA advisory committees and regulatory staff. The limitations of these agents likely reflect the complexity and redundancy of pathways that regulate energy balance, appetitive drives, nutrient absorption and handling, and energy expenditure. Powerful compensatory mechanisms seem to limit the clinical effects of these single-agent and dual-agent drug therapies. Recognizing these limitations, many clinicians and investigators have suggested the need for a broader array of medications to treat obesity that target different components of the weight regulatory machinery and that can be used in combinations tailored to the needs of different patient subgroups. However, this approach is in the earliest stage of development, and there are few clinically relevant predictors of response to weight loss therapies in individual patient subgroups. This review discusses medications that are currently approved by the FDA for treatment of obesity, along with those that are in the later stages of clinical development.

CURRENT CRITERIA FOR USE OF PHARMACOLOGIC THERAPIES FOR OBESITY

Current recommendations for the pharmacologic treatment of obesity limit those therapies to patients with a body mass index (calculated as weight in kilograms divided by the square of height in meters) greater than 30 kg/m^2 or greater than 27 kg/m^2 with significant obesity comorbidities who have previously failed behavioral and lifestyle approaches alone.[10]

The standard FDA benchmark for clinical efficacy of antiobesity drugs has been a loss of initial body weight that is 5% more than that produced by placebo treatment in the same study. However, in clinical practice the most common criterion has been a 1.8-kg (4-pound) weight loss per month for at least 3 months. Maintaining this weight loss after the first 3 months is used as an indication for continued treatment.[11] Although FDA approval and marketing of antiobesity medications is limited to 3 to 24 months, experienced clinicians recognize that for long-term effectiveness, pharmacotherapy needs to be continued indefinitely. These physicians often continue demonstrably effective weight loss medications for as along as they remain effective and well tolerated. The maximal weight loss effects of these drugs are usually observed within the first 6 to 12 months of use, with diminishing additional benefit thereafter. Some regain of the lost weight in the long-term can be expected, although the magnitude of both the initial weight loss and subsequent weight regain varies widely among patients. When these medications induce weight loss, their cessation is almost always associated with rapid regain of the lost weight.[12,13]

PHARMACOLOGIC THERAPIES FOR OBESITY

Medications for the treatment of obesity can be conveniently classified into 4 groups: (1) those that act directly on the GI tract, (2) those that alter gut-brain signaling, (3) those that act directly on the central nervous system (CNS), and (4) formulations that include combinations of different agents.

MEDICATIONS THAT ACT DIRECTLY WITHIN THE GI TRACT

Pancreatic Lipase Inhibitors

Inhibitors of pancreatic and intestinal lipases cause decreased hydrolysis of ingested triglycerides to absorbable fatty acids and monoacylglycerols, thus inducing malabsorption of calorie dense fats.[14] Orlistat is a pancreatic and intestinal lipase inhibitor currently approved by the FDA for the treatment of obesity. It is sold in 2 versions, one available by prescription at a dose of 120 mg 3 times per day (Xenical) and one available over the counter at a reduced dose of 60 mg 3 times per day (Alli). The efficacy of orlistat (120 mg 3 times a day) in reducing weight has been reported in multiple studies, with weight loss averaging 3% to 7% beyond that observed with placebo treatment. This modest weight loss has been shown to be associated with improvement in lipids, insulin resistance, and blood pressure.[15–17] After long-term treatment of up to 4 years, some weight regain has been observed, although orlistat continued to show significantly greater efficacy than placebo.[18,19] Potential side effects of orlistat include flatulence, steatorrhea, fecal incontinence, increased stool frequency, oily rectal discharge, and malabsorption and deficiency of 1 or more fat-soluble vitamins (vitamins A, D, E, and K). In patients receiving chronic orlistat therapy, routine supplementation with a preparation containing these vitamins is advisable. Vitamin D levels should be measured both before and during orlistat therapy, with deficiencies corrected by vigorous supplementation. The recent identification of 13 cases of severe liver injury in patients taking orlistat has generated concern about potential liver toxicity from this agent, and the FDA has added a warning about potential hepatic complications to the labeling. A second lipase inhibitor, cetilistat, is undergoing phase 3 clinical evaluation. The effectiveness of this agent is reputed to be similar to that of orlistat, but early studies suggest that cetilistat is associated with fewer GI side effects.[20]

MEDICATIONS THAT ALTER SIGNALING WITHIN THE GUT-BRAIN AXIS

GLP-1 Agonists

Within the mucosa of the small intestine, specialized enteroendocrine cells release peptides that promote satiety and enhance insulin secretion in response to luminal and circulating nutrients and hormones. Those peptides that enhance insulin secretion in response to nutrient ingestion have been given the name incretins.[21] These peptides exert their effects through interaction with specific receptors on neighboring intestinal epithelial cells, vagal and spinal neurons innervating the gut, or cells in other parts of the body accessed through the portal or peripheral bloodstream. Among these gut-derived peptides, glucagon-like peptide-1 (GLP-1) is the best characterized and currently the most advanced and promising target for antiobesity drug development. GLP-1 is secreted by enteroendocrine L cells in response to luminal nutrients (primarily glucose and other carbohydrates), bile acids, and neural stimulation. These cells are located throughout the small intestine and colon, with highest concentrations in the ileum and proximal colon. Sweet-tasting compounds are among the best-known stimulants of L-cell GLP-1 secretion; these compounds (including sugars) act by binding to specific cell-surface G protein-coupled receptors that activate gustducin-mediated intracellular signaling to stimulate GLP-1 secretion.[22,23] GLP-1 also stimulates insulin secretion in a glucose-dependent manner, inhibits pancreatic glucagon secretion, and has cytoprotective and regenerative actions on pancreatic β cells. It promotes satiety and inhibits food intake, actions that have been associated with demonstrable weight loss. Some studies have also suggested that GLP-1 improves insulin sensitivity.[24]

Exenatide (Byetta), a GLP-1 agonist administered twice daily as a subcutaneous injection at doses of 5 to 10 μg per injection, is currently approved by the FDA for the treatment of type 2 diabetes. Nausea is the most commonly reported side effect. A longer-acting (once-weekly) formulation called Exenatide LAR is undergoing phase 3 clinical evaluation. Liraglutide (Victoza) is a GLP-1 analogue with a longer half-life than exenatide that is also approved by the FDA for the treatment of type 2 diabetes. Its longer half-life allows for once-daily subcutaneous administration at doses between 0.6 and 1.8 mg depending on the glycemic response. A recent, 20-week, double-blind, placebo-controlled, multicenter European trial of liraglutide with an open-label orlistat arm and an 84-week extension open-label follow-up treatment showed superiority of liraglutide over both placebo and orlistat (mean weight loss with various liraglutide doses ranged from 4.8 to 7.2 kg vs 4.1 kg with orlistat and 2.8 kg with placebo).[25] Nausea and vomiting were more common in the liraglutide group, but these symptoms rarely resulted in treatment discontinuation. In this study, liraglutide was also found to improve insulin resistance and prediabetes.[26] However, despite these encouraging results, GLP-1 analogues are not yet approved by the FDA for the treatment of obesity per se. Nonetheless, they are gaining increasing off-label use for this indication, particularly in patients with type 2 diabetes, prediabetes, or other insulin resistance syndromes.

Amylin Analogues

Amylin is a 37-amino acid peptide secreted by the pancreatic β cells primarily in response to meals that augments the effectiveness of insulin in regulating blood glucose. The amylin analogue pramlintide (Symlin) is approved by the FDA as an adjunct to insulin therapy for the treatment of type 2 diabetes. It is administered subcutaneously at a dose of 60 to 120 μg, 2 to 3 times daily before major meals. Pramlintide has been shown to produce more weight loss than exenatide, but side effects, including hypoglycemia, nausea, and vomiting, have limited its off-label use for the treatment of obesity.[27] Clinical studies of pramlintide for the treatment of obesity are ongoing. Early results suggest that there is particular promise in combination therapy with both pramlintide with metreleptin, a synthetic leptin analogue. In this combination, pramlintide seems to enhance leptin responsiveness, and metreleptin is believed to prevent the metabolic adaptation and counterregulatory physiology induced by weight loss generally. In a recent 20-week, phase 2 clinical trial, pramlintide-metreleptin therapy generated an average weight loss of 12.7%.[28]

MEDICATIONS THAT ACT DIRECTLY ON THE CNS

Multiple areas of the brain including the hypothalamus, brainstem, and corticolimbic systems are directly involved in the regulation of food intake, appetite, energy expenditure, and body weight, making them attractive targets for antiobesity drug development. Several agents are available or in clinical development that modify 1 or more of these physiologic and biochemical pathways. The following discussion groups them by the neurotransmitters that they modulate most profoundly.

Dopamine/norepinephrine/serotonin

Phentermine is an amphetamine analogue that activates the sympathetic nervous system through increased norepinephrine and dopamine release, resulting in decreased appetite and increased basal energy expenditure.[29] Phentermine is currently approved by the FDA in 2 formulations: phentermine resin (Ionamin, and others) with available doses of 15 to 30 mg/d, and phentermine·HCl, with available doses of 18.75 to 37.5 mg/d. Both formulations have apparently equivalent clinical effects. Common side effects of phentermine include tachycardia and hypertension; therefore, pulse and blood pressure should be monitored closely after starting this therapy. Although phentermine was a component of the popular phen-fen combination, it has not been associated with carcinoid-like valvular heart disease. Fenfluramine, the other component of this combination, has been shown to be responsible for this adverse effect, and it was removed from the market in 1997.[30] Although phentermine is approved by the FDA for weight loss therapy for only 3 months' use, this limitation likely reflects the prevailing perspective at the time of approval in the late 1950s that medical therapy for obesity was best used as a jump-start for lifestyle modification. With the recognition of the chronic nature of obesity and its pathophysiologic underpinnings, common practice among many obesity medicine specialists is to continue phentermine for as long as it is clinically effective and well tolerated.

Sibutramine (Meridia) is a monoamine reuptake inhibitor of norepinephrine, serotonin, and dopamine that was previously approved by the FDA for the treatment of obesity. At the request of the FDA, this drug was removed from the market in October 2010 after a large, multicenter, long-term, European trial in patients with preexisting cardiovascular disease or type 2 diabetes revealed that subjects in the sibutramine-treated group experienced a significantly higher rate of new cardiovascular events than those in the placebo-treated group.[31,32] These developments have caused reevaluation of the usefulness and safety of monoamine uptake inhibitors for the treatment of patients with obesity, many of whom have cardiovascular disease or diabetes or are at high risk of developing these disorders. As a result, the future of tesofensine, a newer dopamine, norepinephrine, and serotonin reuptake inhibitor that has shown promise in a recent phase 2 clinical trial, is uncertain.[33]

Bupropion is a well-tolerated antidepressant that inhibits reuptake of dopamine and norepinephrine and has been shown to inhibit appetite and food intake in many patients. Bupropion comes in a sustained release (SR) formulation, with doses of 300 to 400 mg per day often effective for the treatment of obesity. A meta-analysis reported 2.77 kg (confidence interval 1.1–4.5 kg) weight loss at 6 to 12 months.[15] Bupropion can decrease the seizure threshold and is therefore contraindicated in patients with known seizure disorders.

Serotonin

The role of serotonin in modulation of food intake is well recognized and has been the bases of the off-label use of fluoxetine (prozac) and sertraline (zoloft), selective serotonin reuptake inhibitors, for the treatment of obesity. Fluoxetine has a good safety profile, but has not been shown as a single agent dosed at 60 mg daily to be more effective than placebo in long-term weight management.[34] Combination therapy with low-dose fluoxetine (10–20 mg per day) and phentermine has been reported to have a greater weight loss effect than treatment with even higher doses of either drug alone.[35]

The identification of several distinct serotonergic (5-hydroxytryptamine [5-HT]) receptors and identification of the 5-HT_2c receptor as the primary mediator of the anorexiant effects of serotonin has allowed specific targeting of these receptors to reduce food intake. Because other 5-HT receptors (especially 5-HT_{2B}) have been shown to be responsible for the cardiac valvular side effects of fenfluramine, more selective receptor targeting avoids the severe side effects that necessitated the withdrawal of fenfluramine (and dexfenfluramine) from the market.[30]

Lorcaserin is a structural analogue of dexfenfluramine that selectively activates 5-HT_2c serotonergic receptors with little or no activation of the 5-HT_2b receptor.[36] In recent phase 3 clinical trials, lorcaserin at 10 mg twice daily for 1 year induced approximately 3.5% more weight loss than that seen in placebo controls.[37] Lorcaserin-treated patients exhibited no increased risk of cardiac valvulopathy. However, because of ongoing concerns about risk-benefit profile, in December 2010 the FDA denied approval of this agent pending a more extensive safety evaluation. The future of this agent is therefore in doubt. However, if it is ultimately approved it will be an attractive candidate for use in combination with phentermine, to reproduce the synergistic weight loss effect shown by combining fenfluramine with phentermine (phen-fen).

COMBINATION THERAPIES

Because of the complexity and redundancy of the regulatory pathways that regulate eating behavior, nutrient absorption, and energy expenditure, it is unlikely that a single drug will emerge as the silver bullet for the treatment of obesity. The dramatic and durable weight loss in response to Roux-en-Y gastric bypass and other types of bariatric surgery likely results from the ability of these operations to influence multiple relevant pathways simultaneously. Combinations of pharmacologic therapies have shown promise in achieving synergistic results. Two centrally acting anticonvulsants that act through the modulation of brain γ-aminobutyric acid pathways (zonisamide and topiramate) and the opioid antagonist naltrexone have emerged as valuable contributors to effective combinations.

Phentermine/topiramate (Qnexa)

This slow-release formulation capitalizes on the apparent synergy between these 2 medications, using smaller doses of each one (15 mg of phentermine and 92 mg of topiramate) than when they are used alone. This approach has the benefit of reducing the risk of side effects from each agent. Although 3 phase 3 randomized controlled trials of Qnexa have reported substantial benefit (average 9% weight loss over placebo controls) and a good safety protocol, this combination therapy was not approved by the FDA in 2010 because of concern about the risk of side effects when the drug is prescribed widely across the population.[38] Both phentermine and topiramate are approved by the FDA as single agents (topiramate is approved for treatment of seizures and migraines). Many obesity medicine specialists use them in combination, starting with a low dose of each agent (eg, topiramate at 25 mg/d and phentermine at 7.5–15 mg/d) and escalating the dose slowly to limit the risk of side effects.

Bupropion/naltrexone (Contrave)

This combination is believed to synergistically enhance the release of the anorexiant neuropeptide α-melanocyte-stimulating hormone, which signals through the melanocortin-4 receptor, a central regulator of food intake.[39,40] Three phase 3 clinical trials have shown that Contrave-32 (360 mg bupropion SR and 32 mg naltrexone SR) generate an average weight loss of approximately 5%. The most frequently reported side effects associated with this combination were nausea, headache, constipation, dizziness, vomiting, and dry mouth, which were more frequently reported with this combination compared with placebo.[41,42] Because of concern about potential cardiovascular side effects, the FDA denied approval of this agent in January 2011 pending a more extensive safety evaluation. However, as with Qnexa, both components of Contrave are available for use as individual agents. Although naltrexone alone seems to promote little weight loss in most patients, the data from the Contrave trials suggest that it can add to the efficacy of bupropion, which has some efficacy as a stand-alone agent. Important caveats in the use of these agents are that bupropion is contraindicated in patients at increased risk of seizures, and naltrexone should not be used in patients who are concomitantly taking narcotic analgesics, either by prescription or illicitly.

Bupropion Plus Zonisamide (Empatic)

Zonisamide is another anticonvulsant that has shown promise for the treatment of obesity. Used as a stand-alone agent in doses up to 600 mg/d, it has been studied in combination with bupropion in a recent phase 2 clinical trial. In this trial, the combination of zonisamide, at doses of 120 to 360 mg/d and 280 to 360 mg/d bupropion generated significant weight loss.[9] Phase 3 clinical trials are planned for this promising combination. Because both components of the combination are available for use as individual agents, many experienced clinicians have prescribed them together to achieve the apparent benefits of the combination.

FUTURE CONSIDERATIONS

Obesity results from the effect of the modern, highly obesogenic environment acting on individuals who are genetically and biologically susceptible to its effects. The changed environment, which includes changes in the chemical composition of food, a reduced need for physical activity, and a variety of enhanced stressors, seems to disrupt many of the physiologic regulatory pathways controlling food-intake behavior, nutrient handling, and energy expenditure so as to alter the body's energy storage set point. The interplay between these regulatory systems and the altered environment leads to excess fat storage and obesity and its myriad metabolic and physical consequences.[43] Because of these complex interactions, it is likely that no single drug or device fully reverses the pathophysiologic processes underlying obesity. Combinations of drugs, targeted nutritional manipulations, and other approaches (eg, endoscopic surgery, endoscopic devices, and minimally invasive surgery) likely offer an effective and safe alternative to current GIWLS procedures. Because these new approaches are less invasive and likely have an improved risk profile, they should be more widely applicable to the large and diverse population of individuals with obesity and its many complications. Combination therapies have several natural advantages, including improved efficacy, diminished risk, and ability to customize combinations for different subgroups of patients. Because of these benefits, such approaches hold the promise of having a significant effect on the profound public health challenge created by the current obesity epidemic.

REFERENCES

1. Flegal KM, Carroll MD, Ogden CL, et al. Prevalence and trends in obesity among US adults, 1999–2008. JAMA 2010;303(3):235–41.
2. Guh DP, Zhang W, Bansback N, et al. The incidence of co-morbidities related to obesity and overweight: a systematic review and meta-analysis. BMC Public Health 2009;9:88.
3. Ogden CL, Carroll MD, Curtin LR, et al. Prevalence of overweight and obesity in the United States, 1999–2004. JAMA 2006;295(13):1549–55.
4. Nguyen NT, Magno CP, Lane KT, et al. Association of hypertension, diabetes, dyslipidemia, and metabolic syndrome with obesity: findings from the National Health and Nutrition Examination Survey, 1999 to 2004. J Am Coll Surg 2008; 207(6):928–34.
5. Rose G. Strategy of prevention: lessons from cardiovascular disease. Br Med J (Clin Res Ed) 1981;282(6279):1847–51.
6. Wing RR. Long-term effects of a lifestyle intervention on weight and cardiovascular risk factors in individuals with type 2 diabetes mellitus: four-year results of the look AHEAD trial. Arch Intern Med 2010;170(17):1566–75.
7. Sjostrom L, Narbro K, Sjostrom CD, et al. Effects of bariatric surgery on mortality in Swedish obese subjects. N Engl J Med 2007;357(8):741–52.
8. Ogden CL, Yanovski SZ, Carroll MD, et al. The epidemiology of obesity. Gastroenterology 2007;132(6):2087–102.
9. Witkamp RF. Current and future drug targets in weight management. Pharm Res 2010. [Epub ahead of print].
10. Clinical Guidelines on the Identification. Evaluation, and Treatment of Overweight and Obesity in Adults–The Evidence Report. National Institutes of Health. Obes Res 1998;6(Suppl 2):51S–209S.
11. Kaplan LM. Pharmacologic therapies for obesity. Gastroenterol Clin North Am 2010;39(1):69–79.
12. Padwal R, Li SK, Lau DC. Long-term pharmacotherapy for obesity and overweight. Cochrane Database Syst Rev 2003;4:CD004094.
13. Bray GA, Greenway FL. Pharmacological treatment of the overweight patient. Pharmacol Rev 2007;59(2):151–84.
14. Padwal RS, Majumdar SR. Drug treatments for obesity: orlistat, sibutramine, and rimonabant. Lancet 2007;369(9555):71–7.
15. Li Z, Maglione M, Tu W, et al. Meta-analysis: pharmacologic treatment of obesity. Ann Intern Med 2005;142(7):532–46.
16. Hutton B, Fergusson D. Changes in body weight and serum lipid profile in obese patients treated with orlistat in addition to a hypocaloric diet: a systematic review of randomized clinical trials. Am J Clin Nutr 2004;80(6):1461–8.
17. Franz MJ, VanWormer JJ, Crain AL, et al. Weight-loss outcomes: a systematic review and meta-analysis of weight-loss clinical trials with a minimum 1-year follow-up. J Am Diet Assoc 2007;107(10):1755–67.
18. Padwal R, Li SK, Lau DC. Long-term pharmacotherapy for obesity and overweight. Cochrane Database Syst Rev 2004;3:CD004094.
19. Padwal R, Li SK, Lau DC. Long-term pharmacotherapy for overweight and obesity: a systematic review and meta-analysis of randomized controlled trials. Int J Obes Relat Metab Disord 2003;27(12):1437–46.

20. Kopelman P, Groot Gde H, Rissanen A, et al. Weight loss, HbA1c reduction, and tolerability of cetilistat in a randomized, placebo-controlled phase 2 trial in obese diabetics: comparison with orlistat (Xenical). Obesity (Silver Spring) 2010;18(1): 108–15.
21. Cummings DE, Overduin J. Gastrointestinal regulation of food intake. J Clin Invest 2007;117(1):13–23.
22. Theodorakis MJ, Carlson O, Michopoulos S, et al. Human duodenal enteroendocrine cells: source of both incretin peptides, GLP-1 and GIP. Am J Physiol Endocrinol Metab 2006;290(3):E550–9.
23. Jang HJ, Kokrashvili Z, Theodorakis MJ, et al. Gut-expressed gustducin and taste receptors regulate secretion of glucagon-like peptide-1. Proc Natl Acad Sci U S A 2007;104(38):15069–74.
24. Hansotia T, Maida A, Flock G, et al. Extrapancreatic incretin receptors modulate glucose homeostasis, body weight, and energy expenditure. J Clin Invest 2007; 117(1):143–52.
25. Astrup A, Rossner S, Van Gaal L, et al. Effects of liraglutide in the treatment of obesity: a randomised, double-blind, placebo-controlled study. Lancet 2009; 374(9701):1606–16.
26. Cummings BP, Stanhope KL, Graham JL, et al. Chronic administration of the glucagon-like peptide-1 analog, liraglutide, delays the onset of diabetes and lowers triglycerides in UCD-T2DM rats. Diabetes 2010;59(10):2653–61.
27. Singh-Franco D, Robles G, Gazze D. Pramlintide acetate injection for the treatment of type 1 and type 2 diabetes mellitus. Clin Ther 2007;29(4):535–62.
28. Roth JD, Roland BL, Cole RL, et al. Leptin responsiveness restored by amylin agonism in diet-induced obesity: evidence from nonclinical and clinical studies. Proc Natl Acad Sci U S A 2008;105(20):7257–62.
29. Halford JC, Boyland EJ, Blundell JE, et al. Pharmacological management of appetite expression in obesity. Nat Rev Endocrinol 2010;6(5):255–69.
30. Connolly HM, Crary JL, McGoon MD, et al. Valvular heart disease associated with fenfluramine-phentermine. N Engl J Med 1997;337(9):581–8.
31. Wadden TA, Berkowitz RI, Womble LG, et al. Randomized trial of lifestyle modification and pharmacotherapy for obesity. N Engl J Med 2005;353(20):2111–20.
32. James WP, Caterson ID, Coutinho W, et al. Effect of sibutramine on cardiovascular outcomes in overweight and obese subjects. N Engl J Med 2010;363(10): 905–17.
33. Astrup A, Madsbad S, Breum L, et al. Effect of tesofensine on bodyweight loss, body composition, and quality of life in obese patients: a randomised, double-blind, placebo-controlled trial. Lancet 2008;372(9653):1906–13.
34. Goldstein DJ, Rampey AH Jr, Enas GG, et al. Fluoxetine: a randomized clinical trial in the treatment of obesity. Int J Obes Relat Metab Disord 1994;18(3):129–35.
35. Anchors M. Fluoxetine is a safer alternative to fenfluramine in the medical treatment of obesity. Arch Intern Med 1997;157(11):1270.
36. Smith SR, Prosser WA, Donahue DJ, et al. Lorcaserin (APD356), a selective 5-HT(2C) agonist, reduces body weight in obese men and women. Obesity (Silver Spring) 2009;17(3):494–503.
37. Smith SR, Weissman NJ, Anderson CM, et al. Multicenter, placebo-controlled trial of lorcaserin for weight management. N Engl J Med 2010;363(3):245–56.
38. Ioannides-Demos LL, Piccenna L, McNeil JJ. Pharmacotherapies for obesity: past, current, and future therapies. J Obes 2011;2011:179674.
39. Cone RD. Anatomy and regulation of the central melanocortin system. Nat Neurosci 2005;8(5):571–8.

40. Nicholson JR, Peter JC, Lecourt AC, et al. Melanocortin-4 receptor activation stimulates hypothalamic brain-derived neurotrophic factor release to regulate food intake, body temperature and cardiovascular function. J Neuroendocrinol 2007;19(12):974–82.
41. Greenway FL, Fujioka K, Plodkowski RA, et al. Effect of naltrexone plus bupropion on weight loss in overweight and obese adults (COR-I): a multicentre, randomised, double-blind, placebo-controlled, phase 3 trial. Lancet 2010;376(9741): 595–605.
42. Wadden TA, Foreyt JP, Foster GD, et al. Weight loss with naltrexone SR/bupropion SR combination therapy as an adjunct to behavior modification: the COR-BMOD trial. Obesity (Silver Spring) 2011;19(1):110–20.
43. Froguel P, Blakemore AI. The power of the extreme in elucidating obesity. N Engl J Med 2008;359(9):891–3.

Bariatric Surgical Anatomy and Mechanisms of Action

Daniel M. Herron, MD*, Ramin Roohipour, MD

KEYWORDS

- Bariatric surgery • Anatomy • Endoscopy • Gastric bypass
- Adjustable gastric band • Sleeve gastrectomy
- Biliopancreatic diversion with duodenal switch

Bariatric surgery is becoming increasingly common such that it is now the second most common abdominal procedure in the United States.[1] Estimates suggest that about 220,000 patients underwent bariatric surgery in 2009.[2] It stands to follow that gastroenterologists will be called on with increasing frequency to perform endoscopic procedures on bariatric patients. In order for the endoscopist to diagnose and treat the bariatric patient, it is critical to have a thorough understanding of the anatomy of the different bariatric procedures, both those in current use and those no longer performed.[3] This article reviews the most commonly encountered bariatric procedures in the United States, and the associated surgical anatomy. In addition, current understanding of the mechanisms of action of these procedures is discussed.

TRADITIONAL CLASSIFICATION OF BARIATRIC PROCEDURES

Historically, bariatric operations have been classified into 1 of 3 categories: restrictive, malabsorptive, or combined.[4] The restrictive category has traditionally included operations such as vertical banded gastroplasty (VBG) that served to limit the functional volume of the stomach and induce weight loss by restricting oral intake.[5] Malabsorptive operations were considered to be those that limited digestion and absorption by rerouting the intestinal path taken by food and digestive enzymes, such as the no longer performed jejunoileal bypass. Combined operations were considered to be those that had elements of both restriction and malabsorption,

---

Disclosures: Dr Herron receives a restricted educational grant from Covidien Inc. Dr Roohipour has no conflicts of interest to disclose.

Department of Surgery, Mount Sinai School of Medicine, 1 Gustave L. Levy Place, #1259, New York, NY 10029, USA
* Corresponding author.
E-mail address: daniel.herron@mountsinai.org

Gastrointest Endoscopy Clin N Am 21 (2011) 213–228
doi:10.1016/j.giec.2011.02.005
giendo.theclinics.com

such as the Roux-en-Y gastric bypass and biliopancreatic diversion with duodenal switch (BPD-DS).

These distinctions are becoming less relevant as more about the endocrine and metabolic effects of bariatric procedures is learned.[6,7] For example, it is commonly noted that gastric bypass patients have an early reduction in appetite starting in the immediate postoperative phase that is unrelated to mechanical filling of the gastric pouch.[8] In addition, patients with type 2 diabetes mellitus undergoing gastric bypass experience an immediate improvement in their glucose metabolism that appears to be unrelated to weight loss.[9] These and other findings suggest that mechanical restriction and malabsorption may be less relevant than the substantial endocrine and metabolic effects that occur after surgery. Thus, the historically useful categorization of procedures as restrictive or malabsorptive is becoming less relevant.

Today, the most commonly performed bariatric operations in the United States include the Roux-en-Y gastric bypass, the laparoscopic adjustable gastric band, the vertical sleeve gastrectomy, and BPD-DS. In this review of bariatric anatomy and mechanisms of action, the authors focus individually on each of these procedures.

HISTORICAL GASTRIC BYPASS (BILLROTH II LOOP TECHNIQUE)

Gastric bypass was first used to treat severe obesity in the 1960s.[10–12] Initially, the operation involved the creation of a gastric pouch by firing a multirow surgical stapler horizontally across the mid-upper stomach. This horizontally oriented pouch included the entire gastric fundus along its upper edge and was bound inferiorly by the horizontal staple line (**Fig. 1**). The pouch was anastomosed in an end-to-side manner to a loop of jejunum in manner of a Billroth type II anastomosis. With this early configuration, as with current operations, the lower stomach—generally referred to as the gastric remnant, or bypassed stomach—was completely excluded from the food path. The gastric remnant emptied its mucus and gastric secretions into the duodenum, where it intermixed with bile and pancreatic secretions before passing into the proximal jejunum, also referred to as the afferent limb.

In the Billroth II type anatomy there is a single anastomosis, the gastrojejunostomy. Ingested food leaving the gastric pouch joins with the bile and pancreatic secretions immediately after passing through this anastomosis. The food continues into the efferent limb of the jejunum toward the ileum. It should be emphasized that the terms "afferent limb" and "efferent limb" refer expressly to the loop gastric bypass; these terms should be strictly avoided when describing the anatomy of the Roux-en-Y gastric bypass.

In the early days of bariatric surgery, loop gastric bypass anatomy was preferred because it required only one anastomosis rather than the two required in Roux-en-Y gastric bypass and was felt to be technically easier to perform. However, this anatomy brings the flow of bile and pancreatic juice into contact with the gastric pouch.[13] Without the protective valve action of the pylorus, the pouch is exposed to bile and the patient is at risk for bile reflux gastritis or esophagitis, which can be challenging to treat. In addition, it may in fact be more technically difficult to bring a loop of small intestine to the very uppermost portion of the obese abdomen rather than the single limb of a Roux. For these reasons, the loop gastric bypass has been nearly universally abandoned in favor of the Roux-en-Y gastric bypass.

ROUX-EN-Y GASTRIC BYPASS

The Roux-en-Y operation is named after César Roux, a Swiss surgeon who developed a Y-shaped intestinal reconstruction to decompress an obstructed stomach

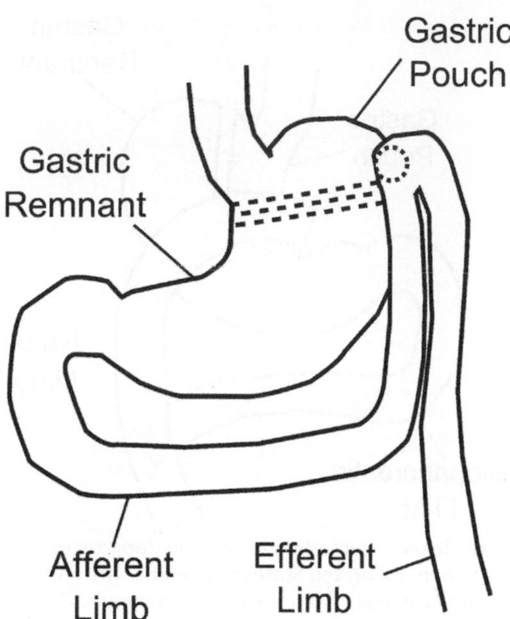

Fig. 1. Loop (Billroth II type) gastric bypass. Of historical relevance, this procedure is no longer performed. The gastric pouch is horizontally oriented, and remains in continuity with the gastric remnant. The jejunum proximal to the gastrojejunostomy is referred to as the afferent limb whereas the distal jejunum is the efferent limb. This terminology is not used when referring to a Roux-en-Y gastric bypass. (*Courtesy of* Daniel M. Herron, © 2010; with permission.)

in 1892.[14] This procedure was first applied to the gastric bypass operation in the 1970s in hopes of eliminating the risk of bile reflux and minimizing tension on the gastrojejunostomy.[15] Over the past two decades, the Roux-en-Y gastric bypass has become the most commonly performed bariatric procedure in the United States (**Fig. 2**).[2]

In the Roux-en-Y gastric bypass the jejunum is typically divided approximately 40 to 100 cm distal to the ligament of Treitz.[16] The distal end is brought up to the stomach pouch and is referred to as the Roux limb, or the alimentary limb, because food but no gastric, bile, or pancreatic secretions passes through this segment. The proximal divided side of the small bowel transmits gastric secretions along with the bile and pancreatic juice, and is thus referred to as the biliopancreatic limb.

The current Roux-en-Y gastric bypass is different from the operations of the 1960s and 1970s in several significant ways. The gastric pouch has evolved to become very small, generally 30 mL in volume or less.[17] Care is taken to completely exclude the fundus from the pouch, to minimize both its volume and the amount of acid-secreting mucosa contained within.

Variation in the technique of pouch formation exists. Some surgeons create a tall, narrow pouch based on the lesser curvature. To accomplish this, the linear surgical stapler is fired transversely across the lesser curvature, approximately 4 to 6 cm distal to the gastroesophageal junction. After this transverse firing, several additional firings are run vertically, parallel to lesser curvature, completely excluding the fundus and forming the left side of the pouch. Other surgeons create a more transversely oriented pouch by firing the stapler several times just underneath the gastroesophageal

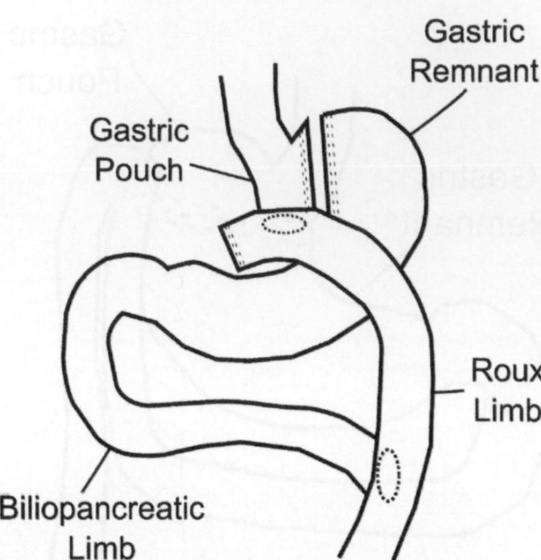

Fig. 2. Roux-en-Y gastric bypass. Typically performed laparoscopically, this is the most common bariatric operation in the United States at present. The gastric pouch is small, vertically oriented, and completely divided from the gastric remnant. Gastric secretions, bile and pancreatic juice flows through the biliopancreatic limb, while ingested food passes through the Roux limb. The bowel distal to the lower anastomosis is referred to as the common channel. (*Courtesy of* Daniel M. Herron, © 2010; with permission.)

junction.[18] Still others create a pouch so small as to be referred to as a "virtual pouch," functionally similar to an esophagojejunostomy.

Another significant difference in the modern gastric bypass is a direct result of the newer staplers. Surgeons of the 1970s and 1980s used a linear stapler that formed a double row of staggered titanium staples (Covidien TA-90; Covidien, Mansfield, MA, USA). While this created a compartmentalized stomach, the pouch and gastric remnant remained in direct continuity. Because of unacceptably high rates of gastric pouch-to-gastric remnant fistula formation across the staple line (gastrogastric fistula), the stapler was modified to lay down 2 additional rows of staggered staples, for a total of 4 rows (TA-90B; Covidien). Some surgeons applied this stapler to the tissue twice, effectively placing 8 rows of superimposed staples. Current staplers function quite differently in that they form 2 triple rows of staples, then divide the tissue down the middle with a cutting blade, creating a "divided pouch" that is fully separated from the gastric remnant. Although there was initial concern that this might lead to an increased staple line leak rate, this has not occurred.[19]

LAPAROSCOPIC APPROACH

In 2010, the majority of Roux-en-Y gastric bypass operations are performed through a laparoscopic approach.[20] The use of 5 to 7 small incisions rather than a single 15- to 30-cm vertical midline incision generally results in fewer wound-related complications, less postoperative pain, and a shorter convalescence.[21] Regardless of whether the surgical approach is laparoscopic or open, the resultant internal visceral anatomy is the same.

The overwhelming majority of laparoscopic linear staplers in current use divide the tissue after it has been stapled. In a laparoscopic gastric bypass, the pouch is most commonly created using a surgical stapler that fires 3 rows of staples on the proximal side and another 3 rows of staples on the distal side, then cuts the intervening tissue. This action creates a fully divided gastric pouch, in contradistinction to earlier approaches in which staples were applied but the stomach tissue was not divided. The use of a fully divided pouch has resulted in a decreased risk of fistula formation between pouch and remnant.[22–24]

The gastric pouch created in a laparoscopic procedure is quite small, generally 15 to 30 mL in volume. On endoscopy, the pouch is entered immediately distal to the gastroesophageal junction. The pouch may have several different configurations, and may be long and narrow or short and wide. Regardless of the configuration of the pouch, the gastrojejunostomy anastomosis should be easily visible within several centimeters of the gastroesophageal junction.

The gastrojejunostomy may be formed using any number of different surgical techniques. Many surgeons prefer using a circular stapler in which 2 concentric rows of titanium staples are fired to connect the end of the pouch to the side of the Roux limb. If this method has been used then it is expected that some staples may be visible internally on endoscopy. Some surgeons prefer the use of a linear cutting stapler to anastomose the side of the stomach pouch to the side of the Roux limb. The remaining enterotomy through which the linear stapler has been inserted is then closed, generally using absorbable suture material. Other surgeons prefer a more traditional surgical technique in which 2 layers of absorbable or permanent sutures are placed using a standard hand-suturing technique.

Regardless of technique, most anastomotic approaches result in and end-to-side type connection, whereby the distal end of the gastric pouch is connected to the side of the Roux limb. On endoscopy, 2 passages into small bowel should be clearly visible immediately beyond the gastrojejunostomy. One limb of bowel will end blindly within several centimeters, while the other will pass down toward the distal anastomosis (jejunojejunostomy). The distance from the gastrojejunostomy to the distal anastomosis is variable but is typically between 40 and 100 cm, generally beyond the reach of a typical upper endoscope.

ALTERNATIVE TYPES OF GASTRIC BYPASS

Although the vast majority of gastric bypasses are performed using the generally accepted techniques described thus far, some surgeons prefer alternative operations. One such example is the so-called mini-gastric bypass, which is a laparoscopic version of the Billroth II loop-type gastric bypasses.[25] Proponents of this approach suggest that it is technically easier to perform because there is only a single gastrointestinal anastomosis to create. Although acceptable weight loss results have been reported with this operation, surgeons' concern regarding the potential for bile reflux gastritis or esophagitis has kept this technique from becoming widespread.[26]

LAPAROSCOPIC ADJUSTABLE GASTRIC BAND

The laparoscopic adjustable gastric band (LAGB) has been available outside the United States since the 1990s and has been performed in the United States since 2001 (**Fig. 3**).[27] At present the Food and Drug Administration (FDA) has approved two different brands; the LAP-BAND device is manufactured by Allergan Inc (Irvine, CA, USA) while the Realize band is made by Ethicon Inc (Somerville, NJ, USA). Although there are minor differences in design between the two brands, they function very similarly within the human body. Weight loss after LAGB placement is variable, but has been reported to range from 40% up to 70% of initial excess body weight.[28,29]

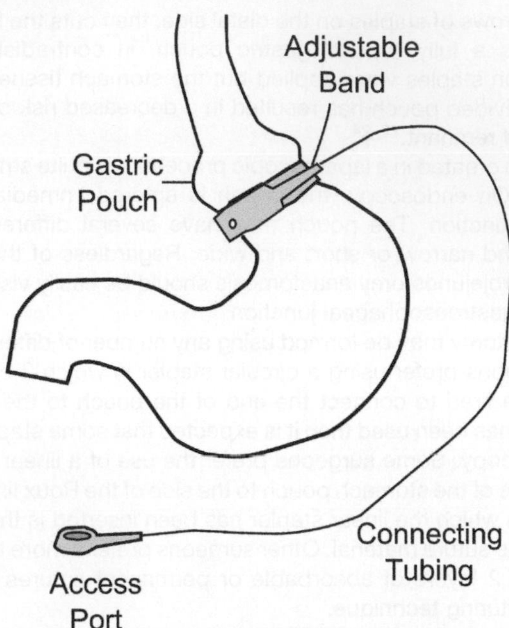

Fig. 3. Laparoscopic adjustable gastric band. A rigid band with an inflatable balloon lining the inner aspect is placed around the upper stomach. The band can be tightened by injecting saline into the subcutaneous access port. Most surgeons in the United States secure the band anteriorly by using 2 to 5 sutures to imbricate the stomach over the band, not shown in this diagram. (*Courtesy of* Daniel M. Herron, © 2010; with permission.)

The bands are placed via laparoscopic surgical approach, around the stomach immediately beneath the gastroesophageal junction, and locked in place using a buckle-type fastener. Anteriorly, the band is fixed in position by imbricating the body of the stomach upward over the band and suturing the fold back to the upper stomach. Some surgeons believe that anterior fixation is unnecessary and omit this step. Posteriorly, the band is held in position by retroperitoneal tissue because the band is placed above the peritoneal reflection of the lesser sac.

The inner surface of the band consists of a saline-filled silicone balloon that is connected, via internal silicone tubing, to a subcutaneous access port. The port, generally located on the anterior abdominal wall near the subcostal, subxiphoid, or periumbilical area, is accessed percutaneously with a noncoring Huber needle. Injecting saline inflates the band and increases restriction whereas removing saline does the opposite.

The band and access port are radio-opaque and are clearly visualized on a plain radiograph of the upper abdomen.[30] A normal band will appear immediately below the gastroesophageal junction, and will be oriented horizontally or with the left side slightly higher than the right (up to about 30° from the horizontal). If the band appears vertical, or with the left side lower than the right, this may suggest that the band has slipped down on the stomach or that part of the stomach has abnormally prolapsed up through the band, commonly referred to as a "band slip."[31]

Because the band is placed around the serosal surface of the stomach, it should not be directly visible on endoscopy. Located immediately beyond the gastroesophageal junction, the band may be appreciated as an extraluminal constriction. Although it is generally possible to pass the endoscope through the lumen of the band into the main stomach compartment, this may be difficult or impossible depending on the tightness of the band, the caliber of the endoscope, and the presence of inflammation or edema in the gastric tissue. Once past the band, the endoscope can be retroflexed to provide a clear view of the band's position.

If any plastic or rubber portion of the band is visible on endoscopy, this represents a highly abnormal finding that necessarily implies that the device has eroded through the full thickness of the esophagus or stomach.[32] Erosion may occur because of surgical trauma at the time of initial operation or as a result of infection or abscess formation immediately adjacent to the band, resulting in inflammation and breakdown of the gastric wall. In general, erosion begins in one small area of the band and gradually enlarges. Erosion may progress to the point where the entire gastric portion of the band becomes intraluminal. Eroded bands are typically removed via a laparoscopic surgical approach. Several reports describe removal of such eroded bands through an endoscopic approach, although a surgical procedure is still required to remove the access port component.[33,34]

Whereas erosion is fairly straightforward to diagnose on endoscopy, band slippage may be a more difficult assessment. If the mucosa is intact but the pouch seems excessively large or the constricted area particularly low on the stomach, this may represent a gastric prolapse or band slip.

Adjustable gastric bands should not be confused with nonadjustable gastric bands, which were used in the 1970s and 1980s and have since fallen into disfavor.[35] These bands were strips of polypropylene mesh that were surgically wrapped around the mid-portion of the stomach and sutured in place. Similarly, the adjustable gastric band is distinct from the VBG, referred to by many laypeople as a "stomach stapling."[36,37] In the VBG a surgical stapler is fired parallel to the lesser curvature to create a narrow pouch similar to that of a gastric bypass. The distal portion of the pouch is constricted by a nonadjustable ring of either polypropylene mesh or silastic tubing. Although popular in the 1980s, the VBG has also fallen out of use because of the difficulty in performing it laparoscopically and its poor long-term weight loss results.[5] Most VBGs were performed using staplers that did not divide the gastric tissue after stapling; as a result, gastric pouch-to-remnant fistula formation is a not uncommon finding.

BILIOPANCREATIC DIVERSION WITH DUODENAL SWITCH

BPD-DS is the only bariatric operation in common use where intestinal malabsorption plays a significant role in weight loss (**Fig. 4**). The operation was first performed in 1988 by two independent groups led by Dr Douglas Hess in Ohio and Dr Picard Marceau in Canada.[38,39] BPD-DS provides better weight loss and comorbidity resolution than any other bariatric procedure.[40] However, these benefits come at the cost of higher morbidity and mortality as well as significant side effects such as diarrhea, excessive flatus, changes in body odor, and other quality-of-life issues.[41,42] Because of its increased technical complexity and potential for complications, the BPD-DS (and its related operation, the BPD without duodenal switch) has not achieved widespread acceptance in the United States, although it is commonly performed in Canada and Italy.

The BPD-DS includes both restrictive and malabsorptive components. Restriction is incurred by a sleeve gastrectomy, sometimes referred to as a vertical sleeve gastrectomy, in which the greater curvature or left side of the stomach is surgically removed. The surgeon accomplishes this resection by serially firing a linear stapler, starting at a point about 5 to 6 cm to the left of the pylorus along the greater curvature. The staple line continues vertically upward, roughly paralleling the lesser curvature, until the

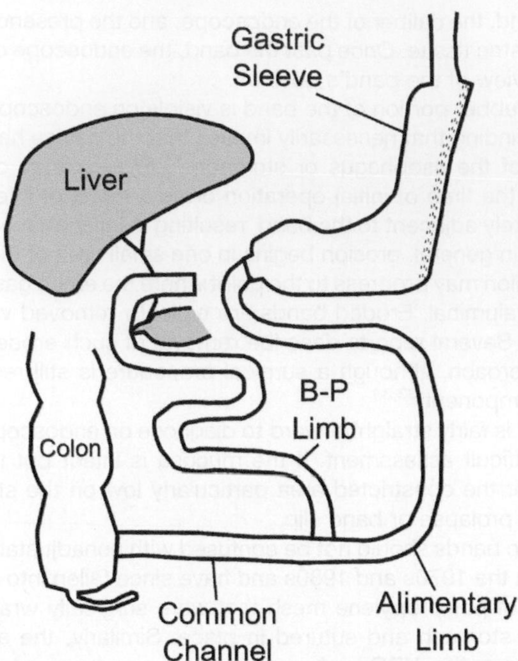

Fig. 4. Biliopancreatic diversion with duodenal switch (BPD-DS). The left side of the stomach is resected, forming a sleeve gastrectomy. The duodenum is divided just distal to the pylorus and connected to the ileum. The remainder of the duodenum and jejunum pass only bile and pancreatic juice; this bypassed intestine is referred to as the biliopancreatic (B-P) limb. The only area where ingested food and digestive juices intermix is the common channel, generally the distalmost 50 to 125 cm of ileum. (*Courtesy of* Daniel M. Herron, © 2010; with permission.)

upper edge of the stomach is reached near the angle of His, approximately 1 to 2 cm left of the gastroesophageal junction. The crescent-shaped resected portion of the stomach is then brought out through one the laparoscopic trocar sites.

The diameter of the sleeve gastrectomy is calibrated at the time of surgery by placing an esophageal bougie through the stomach into the pylorus while the stapling is taking place.[43,44] Although some controversy exists as to the optimal size of bougie, most surgeons use one between 32F (11 mm diameter) and 60F (20 mm diameter). Equally important to the bougie size is the extent to which the surgeon “hugs” the stapler to the bougie as the staple line proceeds upwards. It warrants emphasis that the sleeve gastrectomy is unlike gastric bypass in that the excluded portion of the stomach is removed from the body during surgery, rendering this portion of the operation completely irreversible.

The malabsorptive component of the BPD-DS is a result of 2 anatomic changes: first, the overall length of the alimentary limb is decreased. Second, the intermixing of bile and pancreatic juices is limited to the distalmost portion of the alimentary limb, the so-called common channel, generally 50 to 125 cm in length.[45] These changes are achieved using a modified Roux-en-Y anatomy. First, the duodenum is surgically divided with a linear stapler several centimeters distal to the pylorus. Second, the ileum is divided approximately 250 to 300 cm proximal to the ileocecal junction. The distal divided end of the ileum is then anastomosed to the proximal divided duodenum, forming the alimentary limb. The remaining small intestine, containing only bile and pancreatic secretions, is anastomosed in an end-to-side manner to the distal ileum, typically 50 to 125 cm proximal to the ileocecal junction. This final segment of ileum, serving as the lowermost limb of the "Y," is referred to as the common channel, and is where the ingested food finally intermixes with bile and pancreatic juice.

If one follows a hypothetical ingested food particle through BPD-DS anatomy, it passes across the gastroesophageal junction through a long narrow stomach, past the intact pylorus, then immediately into the last 250 cm or so of ileum before reaching the colon. The food does not intermix with bile or pancreatic secretions until it reaches the segment of bowel beyond the distal anastomosis, the common channel. This very limited contact between ingested food and digestive enzymes results in substantial impairment of absorption of both protein and fat.[46] This malabsorption is responsible for the remarkable weight loss seen after BPD-DS, up to 80% of initial excess body weight or more.[40] However, it is also to blame for the nutritional deficiencies, namely hypoalbuminemia and fat-soluble vitamin deficiency.[41] In addition, it results in the soft bowel movements and increased flatus noted by many BPD-DS patients postoperatively, particularly during the early postoperative phase.[47]

On endoscopic evaluation, the stomach will appear to be quite long and narrow. The fundus will be surgically absent. Due to the narrow gastric anatomy, it may be difficult to retroflex the endoscope to obtain a retrograde view of the gastroesophageal junction. However, the narrow caliber of the stomach minimizes bowing of the endoscope and facilitates passage through the intact pylorus. Immediately past the pylorus, the proximal anastomosis, or duodenoileostomy, will be traversed. This anastomosis may have been formed using either a stapled or hand-sewn technique, so the endoscopist may or may not visualize staples on the mucosal surface. The distal anastomosis will be approximately 100 cm further downstream, so is not generally reached on upper endoscopy.

For unclear reasons, the formation of strictures at the duodenoileostomy is exceedingly rare, in contradistinction to gastric bypass whereby stricture rate may be as high as 10% depending on surgical technique.[48,49] However, narrowing of the stomach itself may be noted in the area of the incisura, where the lateral staple line passes closest to the lesser curvature. Such narrowing is exaggerated shortly after surgery, when postsurgical edema is still present, and is commonly responsible for early postoperative nausea and vomiting.[50]

Although patients may complain of reflux-type symptoms after BPD-DS, it should be remembered that most of the acid-producing stomach tissue has been removed.[51] Such symptoms may potentially be caused by stasis of ingested food in the lower esophagus.

SLEEVE GASTRECTOMY

Sleeve gastrectomy as a separate procedure was initially used as the first part of a 2-stage BPD-DS (**Fig. 5**).[52] Early in their experience, surgeons found that gastric bypass and BPD-DS patients with a body mass index (BMI; weight in kilograms divided by height in meters squared, ie, kg/m^2) of greater than 60 suffered from an excessively high rate of technical complications. In an attempt to reduce the complexity of the procedure and minimize its complications, surgeons performed the sleeve gastrectomy as a primary operation, avoiding the more technically complex aspects of the duodenal division and reanastomosis.[53] The goal of sleeve gastrectomy as a "first stage" operation was that it would result in 50 kg or more of weight loss—enough to

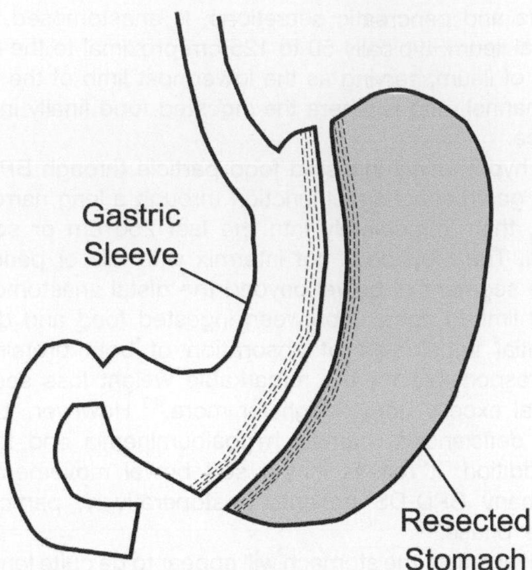

Fig. 5. Sleeve gastrectomy. The left side (greater curvature) of the stomach is resected, leaving a long, narrow stomach based on the lesser curvature. With weight loss and diabetes resolution better than the adjustable gastric band, this operation is rapidly increasing in popularity. (*Courtesy of* Daniel M. Herron, © 2010; with permission.)

significantly reduce the technical complexity of the "second stage" operation that would complete the BPD-DS anatomy.

Investigators discovered that many patients were able to lose enough weight with the sleeve gastrectomy that a second stage was not required; this led to sleeve gastrectomy being used as a primary operation in patients with BMIs well below 60.[43] Later studies found sleeve gastrectomy to result in weight loss and comorbidity resolution somewhere between that of adjustable gastric banding and Roux-en-Y gastric bypass.[54]

The concept of sleeve gastrectomy rapidly grew in popularity, as it had significant appeal to both surgeons and potential patients. The operation seemingly embodied the best aspects of both band and bypass. The weight loss is excellent, typically 50% to 60% of initial excess body weight, and the resolution of diabetes afterwards (70%) significantly exceeds that seen with the gastric band.[55] Unlike the gastric band, there is no implantation of a medical device and no need for postoperative adjustment. Because no bowel is bypassed, the need for nutritional supplementation is significantly less than that in gastric bypass and BPD-DS.

These attributes led to sleeve gastrectomy becoming the fastest-growing bariatric procedure in the United States during the last several years, despite the initial reluctance of many third-party payors to recognize it. Although Medicare has taken the position that sleeve gastrectomy is investigational and therefore not covered, many private insurers have reversed their earlier positions and now consider the sleeve to be a legitimate surgical option.[56] With the operation receiving its own CPT (Current Procedural Terminology) code in 2010, it is anticipated that the general acceptance of the procedure will continue to grow.

Initially, it was felt that sleeve gastrectomy was a purely restrictive operation. However, recent studies have demonstrated multiple biochemical changes postoperatively, resulting in decreased appetite and improvements in glucose metabolism.[57,58]

From an endoscopist's perspective, the internal anatomy of the sleeve gastrectomy is essentially identical to that seen in the gastric portion of the BPD-DS (see earlier discussion). The endoscopist should, however, be aware of the trend toward narrower sleeves. Initially, the sleeves created as part of the BPD-DS were calibrated using a 60F bougie (20 mm diameter). With increasing experience it was found that narrower sleeves resulted in better weight loss.[44] As a result, most surgeons currently use a bougie of 32F to 40F (11–13 mm diameter) to calibrate the sleeve.

OBSOLETE BARIATRIC PROCEDURES AND DEVICES

There are several bariatric procedures that are no longer in use. The jejunoileal bypass is one such procedure that was abandoned more than 20 years ago because of its severe metabolic complications including protein malabsorption, fat-soluble vitamin deficiency, and liver failure.[59] In the jejunoileal bypass the jejunum was divided just distal to the ligament of Treitz and re-anastomosed to the distal ileum, with the intention of causing significant malabsorption. Although this procedure resulted in excellent weight loss, the complications were frequent and severe, and the operation has been completely abandoned.[60] Although most patients who underwent this operation have since had it reversed, the gastroenterologist may occasionally encounter a patient with intact jejunoileal bypass anatomy. Such patients should be referred to a bariatric surgeon for reversal or revision using a safer procedure.

The gastric balloon is an implantable device that was briefly used in the mid-1980s. Developed by 2 gastroenterologists, the device was approved by the FDA in 1985. Consisting of a silicone balloon that was passed into the stomach via an endoscope and inflated, the device was intended to stimulate satiety signals and reduce the functional capacity of the stomach.[61] However, early sham-controlled studies demonstrated poor weight loss outcomes and high rates of complication, including gastric erosion, ulceration, small bowel obstruction, and esophageal laceration.[62] The device was pulled from the market and its FDA approval revoked. At present no gastric balloons are in general clinical use, although several new devices are under investigation as temporary (up to 6 months) weight loss aids.

FUTURE PROCEDURES AND DEVICES

Given the increasing prevalence of Class III obesity and type 2 diabetes mellitus, it can be expected that the interest in new treatments for obesity will continue to grow, in the form of both surgical procedures and medical devices. Several investigational procedures and devices are worth mentioning here, as they may be approved for clinical use in the near future.

Endoscopic Tissue Plication Devices

Several endoscopic devices are currently cleared by the FDA for use in endoluminal tissue apposition. One such device, StomaphyX (Endogastric Solutions, Redmond, WA, USA) endoscopically applies T-fasteners to gastric tissue, while another, g-Prox (USGI, San Clemente, CA, USA) uses pledgeted suture material to plicate tissue. These devices are currently being used, with variable success, to potentially reduce the size of a gastric bypass pouch or gastrojejunostomy.[63,64] These or similar devices may be used for primary gastric reduction procedures in the near future.

Endoscopic Barrier Devices

Endoscopically deployed plastic tubes have been investigated as intestinal mucosal barrier devices. By restricting the contact of ingested food with intestinal mucosa, it is hoped that such devices could result in weight loss and diabetes control. Published rat studies are encouraging, but it is not anticipated that such devices would provide more than temporary therapy.[65]

Gastric Plication Procedures

Surgical plication of the stomach has been used as early as 1989 for antireflux purposes.[66] More recently, plication has been performed via laparoscopic approach to reduce gastric volume and compliance in hopes of achieving lasting weight loss.[67] While the long-term data supporting such procedures are lacking, mid-term excess weight loss of 57% to 62% has been reported.[67,68] Such operations could potentially be performed endoscopically as well as laparoscopically.

Duodenojejunal Bypass

Duodenojejunal bypass may be performed with or without sleeve gastrectomy. Functioning as a hybrid between BPD-DS and gastric bypass, the procedure could potentially combine the best aspects of both operations.[69] Although the operation has been demonstrated to be effective in controlling type 2 diabetes in rats, clinical data for humans, while encouraging, are very limited in volume and regarding length of follow-up.[70,71]

Enteric Electrical Stimulation

Electrical stimulation of the stomach and autonomic nervous system has been studied as early as 2002.[72] Although early studies were optimistic, subsequent investigations have dampened enthusiasm, failing to demonstrate durable weight loss or diabetic control.[73] The 2009 SHAPE trial is the most definitive study of gastric electrical stimulation to date.[74] One hundred and ninety subjects were randomized to gastric electrical stimulation or implantation of the device without stimulation; no difference in weight loss between the groups was found. Some investigators remain hopeful that gastric stimulation, although resulting in minimal weight loss, may improve glycemic control in patients with type 2 diabetes.[75]

SUMMARY

As the incidence of clinically significant obesity, type 2 diabetes, and other weight-related comorbid conditions continues to grow, bariatric interventions are being increasingly used to treat these conditions. With each passing year, the number of bariatric patients with surgically altered gastrointestinal anatomy increases. It is critical that any health care provider, particularly those focusing on the gastrointestinal tract, be knowledgable of the bariatric procedures and familiar with their anatomy. In addition, it seems likely that many future bariatric interventions will be applied endoscopically. Whether gastroenterologists are diagnosing and treating sequelae of bariatric surgery or treating the disease primarily, their involvement in the specialty will undoubtedly grow over the upcoming decade.

REFERENCES

1. Birkmeyer NJ, Dimick JB, Share D, et al. Hospital complication rates with bariatric surgery in Michigan. JAMA 2010;304:435–42.
2. American Society for Metabolic and Bariatric Surgery. Available at: http://www.asmbs.org/Newsite07/media/ASMBS_Metabolic_Bariatric_Surgery_Overview_FINAL_09.pdf. Accessed November 3, 2010.

3. Levitzky BE, Wassef WY. Endoscopic management in the bariatric patient. Curr Opin Gatroenterol 2010;26:632–9.
4. Alverdy JC, Prachand V, Flanagan B, et al. Bariatric surgery: a history of empiricism, a future in science. J Gastrointest Surg 2009;13:465–77.
5. Balsiger BM, Poggio JL, Mai J, et al. Ten and more years after vertical banded gastroplasty as primary operation for morbid obesity. J Gastrointest Surg 2000; 4:598–605.
6. Diniz Mde F, Azeredo Passos VM, Diniz MT. Bariatric surgery and the gut-brain communication—the state of the art three years later. Nutrition 2010;26:925–31.
7. Neary MT, Batterham RL. Gut hormones: implications for the treatment of obesity. Pharmacol Ther 2009;124:44–56.
8. O'Brien PE. Bariatric surgery: mechanisms, indications and outcomes. J Gastroenterol Hepatol 2010;25:1358–65.
9. Pories WJ, Swanson MS, MacDonald KG, et al. Who would have thought it? An operation proves to be the most effective therapy for adult-onset diabetes mellitus. Ann Surg 1995;222:339–50.
10. Mason EE, Ito C. Gastric bypass. Ann Surg 1969;170:329–36.
11. Printen KJ, Mason EE. Gastric surgery for relief of morbid obesity. Arch Surg 1973;106:428–31.
12. Buchwald H. Introduction and current status of bariatric procedures. Surg Obes Relat Dis 2008;4:S1–6.
13. Rucker RD, Chan EK, Horstmann J, et al. Searching for the best weight reduction operation. Surgery 1984;96:624–31.
14. Deitel M. Cesar Roux and his contribution. Obes Surg 2007;17:1277–8.
15. Griffen WO, Young VL, Stevenson CC. A prospective comparison of gastric and jejunoileal bypass procedures for morbid obesity. Ann Surg 1977;186(4): 500–7.
16. Higa KD, Boone KB, Davies OG. Laparoscopic Roux-en-Y gastric bypass for morbid obesity: technique and preliminary results for our first 400 patients. Arch Surg 2000;135:1029–33.
17. Higa KD, Boone KB, Ho T. Complications of the laparoscopic Roux-en-Y gastric bypass: 1040 patients—what have we learned? Obes Surg 2000;10:509–13.
18. Schauer PR, Ikramuddin S, Gourash W, et al. Outcomes after laparoscopic Roux-en-Y gastric bypass for morbid obesity. Ann Surg 2000;232(4):515–29.
19. Patel S, Szomstein S, Rosenthal RJ. Reasons and outcomes of reoperative bariatric surgery for failed and complicated procedures. Obes Surg 2010. [Epub ahead of print].
20. Weight control information network, an information service of the National Institute of Diabetes and Digestive and Kidney Diseases (NIDDK). Available at: http://Win.niddk.nih.gov/publications/gastric.htm. Accessed November 3, 2010.
21. Nguyen NT, Goldman C, Rosenquist CJ, et al. Laparoscopic versus open gastric bypass: a randomized study of outcomes, quality of life, and costs. Ann Surg 2001;234:278–89.
22. Cucchi SG, Pories WJ, MacDonald KG, et al. Gastrogastric fistulas: a complication of divided gastric bypass surgery. Ann Surg 1995;221:387–91.
23. Capella JF, Capella RF. Gastro-gastric fistulas and marginal ulcers in gastric bypass procedures for weight reduction. Obes Surg 1999;9:22–7.
24. Carrodeguas L, Szomstein S, Soto F, et al. Management of gastro-gastric fistulas after divided Roux-en-Y gastric bypass surgery for morbid obesity: analysis of 1292 consecutive patients and review of literature. Surg Obes Relat Dis 2005; 1:467–74.

25. Rutledge R. The mini-gastric bypass: experience with the first 1274 cases. Obes Surg 2001;11:276–80.
26. Johnson WH, Fernandez AZ, Farrell RM, et al. Surgical revision of loop ("mini") gastric bypass procedure: muticenter review of complications and conversions to Roux-en-Y gastric bypass. Surg Obes Relat Dis 2007;3(1):37–41.
27. Rubinstein RB. Laparoscopic adjustable gastric banding at a US center with up to 3-year follow-up. Obes Surg 2002;12(3):380–4.
28. Weichman K, Ren C, Kurian M, et al. The effectiveness of adjustable gastric banding: a retrospective 6-year U.S. follow-up study. Surg Endosc 2011;25(2): 397–403.
29. Boza C, Gamboa C, Awruch D, et al. Laparoscopic Roux-en-Y gastric bypass versus laparoscopic adjustable gastric banding: five years of follow-up. Surg Obes Relat Dis 2010;6:470–5.
30. Weisner W, Schob O, Hauser RS, et al. Adjustable laparoscopic gastric banding in patients with morbid obesity: radiographic management, results and postoperative complications. Radiology 2000;216:389–94.
31. Szucs RA, Turner MA, Kellum JM, et al. Adjustable laparoscopic gastric band for the treatment of morbid obesity: radiographic evaluation. AJR Am J Roentgenol 1998;170(4):993–6.
32. Cherian PT, Goussous G, Ashori F, et al. Band erosion after laparoscopic gastric banding: a retrospective analysis of 865 patients over 5 years. Surg Endosc 2010;24:2031–8.
33. Blero D, Eisendrath P, Vandermeeren A, et al. Endoscopic removal of dysfunctioning bands or rings after restrictive bariatric procedures. Gastrointest Endosc 2010;71:468–74.
34. Neto MP, Ramos AC, Campos JM, et al. Endoscopic removal of eroded adjustable gastric band: lessons learned after 5 years and 78 cases. Surg Obes Relat Dis 2010;6:423–7.
35. Sjoberg EJ, Andersen E, Hoel R, et al. Gastric banding in the treatment of morbid obesity. Factors influencing immediate and long-term results. Acta Chir Scand 1989;155:31–4.
36. MacLean LD, Rhode BM, Shizgal HM. Gastroplasty for obesity. Surg Gynecol Obstet 1981;153:200–8.
37. Eckhout GV, Willbanks OL, Moore JT. Vertical ring gastroplasty for morbid obesity. Five year experience with 1463 patients. Am J Surg 1986;152:713–6.
38. Marceau P, Hould FS, Simard S, et al. Biliopancreatic diversion with duodenal switch. World J Surg 1998;22:947–54.
39. Hess DS, Hess DW. Biliopancreatic diversion with a duodenal switch. Obes Surg 1998;8:267–82.
40. Prachand VN, Davee RT, Alveerdy JC. Duodenal switch provides superior weight loss in the super-obese compared with gastric bypass. Ann Surg 2006;244:611–9.
41. Biertho L, Biron S, Hould FS, et al. Is biliopancreatic diversion with duodenal switch indicated for patients with body mass index <50 kg/m^2? Surg Obes Relat Dis 2010;6:508–14.
42. Hess DS, Hess DW, Oakley RS. The biliopancreatic diversion with the duodenal switch: results beyond 10 years. Obes Surg 2005;15:408–16.
43. Lee CM, Cirangle PT, Jossart GH. Vertical gastrectomy for morbid obesity in 216 patients: report of 2-year results. Surg Endosc 2007;21:1810–6.
44. Parikh M, Gagner M, Heacock L, et al. Laparoscopic sleeve gastrectomy: does bougie size affect mean %EWL? Short term outcomes. Surg Obes Relat Dis 2008;4:528–33.

45. Anthone GJ, Lord RV, DeMeester TR, et al. The duodenal switch operation for the treatment of morbid obesity. Ann Surg 2003;238:618–27.
46. Marceau P, Hould FS, Lebel S, et al. Malabsorptive obesity surgery. Surg Clin North Am 2001;81:1113–27.
47. Wasserberg N, Hamoui N, Petrone P, et al. Bowel habits after gastric bypass versus the duodenal switch operation. Obes Surg 2008;18:1563–6.
48. Buchwald H, Kellogg TA, Leslie DB, et al. Duodenal switch operative mortality and morbidity are not impacted by body mass index. Ann Surg 2008;248:541–8.
49. Ryskina KL, Miller KM, Aisenberg J, et al. Routine management of stricture after gastric bypass and predictors of subsequent weight loss. Surg Endosc 2010;24: 554–60.
50. Lacy A, Obarzabal A, Pando E, et al. Revisional surgery after sleeve gastrectomy. Surg Laparosc Endosc Percutan Tech 2010;20:351–6.
51. Marceau P, Marceau S, Biron S, et al. Long-term experience with duodenal switch in adolescents. Obes Surg 2010;20(12):1609–16.
52. Regan JP, Inabnet WB, Gagner M, et al. Early experience with two-stage laparoscopic Roux-en-Y gastric bypass as an alternative in the super-super obese patient. Obes Surg 2003;13:861–4.
53. Cottam D, Qureshi FG, Mattar SG, et al. Laparoscopic sleeve gastrectomy as an initial weight-loss procedure for high-risk patients with morbid obesity. Surg Endosc 2006;20:859–63.
54. Himpens J, Dobbeleir J, Peeters G. Long-term results of laparoscopic sleeve gastrectomy for obesity. Ann Surg 2010;252:319–24.
55. Abbatini F, Rizzello M, Casella G, et al. Long-term effects of laparoscopic sleeve gastrectomy, gastric bypass, and adjustable gastric banding on type 2 diabetes. Surg Endosc 2010;24:1005–10.
56. Medicare National Coverage Determinations Manual. Available at: https://146.123.140.205/manuals/downloads/ncd103c1_Part2.pdf. Accessed November 3, 2010.
57. Arroyo K, Kini SU, Harvey JE, et al. Surgical therapy for diabesity. Mt Sinai J Med 2010;77:418–30.
58. Gill RS, Birch DW, Shi X, et al. Sleeve gastrectomy and type 2 diabetes mellitus: a systematic review. Surg Obes Relat Dis 2010;6(6):707–13.
59. Brill AB, Sandstead HH, Price R, et al. Changes in body composition after jejunoileal bypass in morbidly obese patients. Am J Surg 1972;123:49–56.
60. Scott HW Jr, Dean RH, Shull HJ, et al. Metabolic complications of jejunoileal bypass operation for morbid obesity. Annu Rev Med 1976;27:397–405.
61. Brody J. Stomach balloon for obesity gains favor amid concerns. New York Times April 29, 1986.
62. Benjamin SB, Maher KA, Carrau EL, et al. Double-blind controlled trial of the Garren-Edwards gastric bubble: an adjunctive treatment for exogenous obesity. Gastroenterology 1988;95:581–8.
63. Horgan S, Jacobsen G, Weiss GD, et al. Incisionless revision of post-Roux-en-Y bypass stomal and pouch dilation: multicenter registry results. Surg Obes Relat Dis 2010;6:290–5.
64. Mikami D, Needleman B, Narula V, et al. Natural orifice surgery: initial US experience utilizing the StomaphyX device to reduce gastric pouches after Roux-en-Y gastric bypass. Surg Endosc 2010;24:223–8.
65. Aguirre V, Stylopoulos N, Grinbaum R, et al. An endoluminal sleeve induces substantial weight loss and normalizes glucose homeostasis in rats with diet-induced obesity. Obesity (Silver Spring) 2008;16:2585–92.

66. Taylor TV, Knox RA, Pullan BR. Vertical gastric plication: an operation for gastro-oesophageal reflux. Ann R Coll Engl 1989;71:31–6.
67. Talebpour M, Amoli BS. Laparoscopic total gastric vertical plication in morbid obesity. J Laparoendosc Adv Surg Tech A 2007;17:793–8.
68. Ramos A, Galvao-Neto M, Galvao M, et al. Laparoscopic greater curvature plication: initial results of an alternative restrictive bariatric procedure. Obes Surg 2010;20(7):913–8.
69. Kasama K, Tagaya N, Kanehira E, et al. Laparoscopic sleeve gastrectomy with duodenojejunal bypass: technique and preliminary results. Obes Surg 2009;19:1341–5.
70. Rubino F, Forgione A, Cummings DE, et al. The mechanism of diabetes after gastrointestinal bypass surgery reveals a role of the proximal small intestine in the pathophysiology of type 2 diabetes. Ann Surg 2006;244:741–9.
71. Cohen RV, Schiavon CA, Pinheiro JS, et al. Duodenal-jejunal bypass for the treatment of type 2 diabetes in patients with body mass index of 22-34 kg/m^2: a report of 22 cases. Surg Obes Relat Dis 2007;3:195–7.
72. Cigaina V. Gastric pacing as therapy for morbid obesity: preliminary results. Obes Surg 2002;12(Suppl 1):12S–6S.
73. Favretti F, DeLuca M, Segato G, et al. Treatment of morbid obesity with the Transcend Implantable Gastric Stimulator (IGS): a prospective survey. Obes Surg 2004;14:666–70.
74. Shikora SA, Bergenstal R, Bessler M, et al. Implantable gastric stimulation for the treatment of clinical severe obesity: results of the SHAPE trial. Surg Obes Relat Dis 2009;5:31–7.
75. Sanmiguel CP, Conklin JL, Cunneen SA, et al. Gastric electrical stimulation with the TANTALUS System in obese type 2 diabetic patients: effect on weight and glycemic control. J Diabetes Sci Technol 2009;3:964–70.

Presurgical Evaluation and Postoperative Care for the Bariatric Patient

Nabil Tariq, MD[a], Bipan Chand, MD[b,*]

KEYWORDS

• Bariatric • Presurgical • Preoperative • Endoscopy • Follow-up

As rates of obesity continue to increase and bariatric surgery becomes increasingly prevalent, more and more specialties encounter bariatric patients during presurgical evaluation and postoperative care. These patients usually have multiple comorbidities and need a comprehensive multisystem evaluation preoperatively and a similar follow-up postoperatively. Bariatric surgery is truly a multidisciplinary management paradigm with involvement of primary care providers, surgeons, bariatricians (medical physicians with expertise in bariatrics), psychologists, nutritionists, and other health care professionals.

The safety of bariatric surgery has gradually improved with the evolution of technique and choice of operations, experience with the procedures, and overall improvement in perioperative care.[1]

Presurgical evaluation is multidisciplinary and can be divided into 3 main components: surgical, medical, and psychological. Unlike most other surgeries, the psychological/behavioral component is very significant because of the lifelong behavior change and commitment that undergoing bariatric surgery requires. The preoperative phase includes not just the evaluation and suitability phase but, equally important, the preparation phase. The preparation phase involves group sessions, individual sessions, seminars, dietary behavior modification, and so on, which are both to test the patients and to make sure that these patients make a well-informed decision if and when they decide to proceed with surgery.

The authors have nothing to disclose.

[a] Flexible Endoscopy and Advanced Laparoscopy, Cleveland Clinic, Cleveland, OH, USA
[b] Bariatric and Metabolic Institute, Cleveland Clinic Main Campus, Mail Code M61, 9500 Euclid Avenue, Cleveland, OH 44195, USA
* Corresponding author.
E-mail address: chandb@ccf.org

Gastrointest Endoscopy Clin N Am 21 (2011) 229–240
doi:10.1016/j.giec.2011.02.010
giendo.theclinics.com
1052-5157/11/$ – see front matter

The eligibility for surgery is based, briefly, on the National Institutes of Health guidelines that suggest that surgery should be considered in patients with a body mass index (BMI, calculated as the weight in kilograms divided by the height in meters squared) of 40 or more without comorbidities or with a BMI of 35 or more with obesity-related comorbidities.[2] Prior upper abdominal, especially gastric, surgery may alter or prohibit bariatric surgery. Prior small bowel surgery may make the procedures with a malabsorptive component (gastric bypass, biliopancreatic diversion with duodenal switch) more difficult or not feasible. Various other conditions such as previous upper abdominal irradiation or liver transplantation may be relative contraindications to bariatric surgery.

There is no distinct age cutoff, but there are concerns in the elderly about increased risk, difficulty in modifying lifestyle, and limited life expectancy that may not be long enough to benefit from the reduction in comorbidities. The concerns remain to be addressed, but many experienced centers operate on patients who are in their 60s and have had good results regarding safety.[1]

PSYCHOLOGICAL AND BEHAVIORAL EVALUATION

The psychological evaluation and preparation is extremely important. A significant proportion of morbidly obese patients have known or undiagnosed psychological illness, such as depression, anxiety, binge eating, or posttraumatic stress disorder. Around half of bariatric patients take psychotropic drugs.[3] Therefore, a thorough evaluation is very important. The social history, life stressors, dietary and weight loss history, and eating disorders of the patient should be evaluated. This screening is very important for long-term success. Most centers look for stability of these conditions and do not attempt to prohibit intervention. Relative contraindications vary from institution to institution but may include smoking, significant alcohol intake, and other substance abuse. Other concerns that may lead to poor long-term success include being consistently abusive to staff, missing multiple appointments, being in an excessive rush to undergo surgery, and significantly gaining weight while in the evaluation process. The relatively long evaluation process of several months with repeated contact with several health care providers helps to tease out some of these issues.

Dietary counseling is initiated preoperatively, is emphasized throughout the preoperative evaluation process, and should be reinforced postoperatively. Dietary indiscretions can lead to persistent postoperative problems such as nausea and pain. The maladaptive eating that may result from these operations may lead to failure of adequate weight loss, overall discontent, and even weight recidivism.

There are not much data to support a preoperative weight loss regimen; however, many believe that losing weight may be very beneficial.[1] We routinely ask all our patients, especially those with a BMI more than 50 to lose 5% to 10% of their excess weight. Losing weight is done with the help of nutritionists and medical bariatricians. Patients may be placed on a modified protein-sparing diet to preserve their protein stores. The weight loss helps decrease visceral fat, making it technically easier to manipulate and retract the liver and small bowel mesentery. This technical ease is especially helpful in the laparoscopic approach and may help reduce complications.[4] Another added benefit is that the patient undergoes a trial of behavior modification and is prepared for the immediate postoperative dietary change. Having bariatric surgery requires a lifelong change in eating habits. Success at a preoperative weight loss regimen may predict who will have a better postoperative weight loss and helps improve patient understanding.

MEDICAL EVALUATION

A comprehensive and thorough medical evaluation is done for perioperative risk stratification and the diagnosis and optimization of comorbid illness. After a thorough history taking and physical examination, routine laboratory work and studies are obtained in all patients as listed in **Table 1**.

There are few medical contraindications to bariatric surgery. More serious or absolute contraindications include incurable cancer, Crohn disease, and severe comorbid conditions that significantly increase perioperative risk such as active angina or decompensated heart failure. AIDS and cirrhosis are generally considered contraindications, but there are reports of safely performing bariatric surgery in human immunodeficiency virus–infected patients who do not have full-blown AIDS and are well controlled with the antiretrovirals.[5] Patients with mild cirrhosis without significant portal hypertension can undergo bariatric surgery, but operative plans may have to be altered, with sleeve gastrectomy being a potential option because both gastric bypass and gastric band surgery require dissection near the esophagogastric junction with the potential for significant bleeding. An overall poor quality of life with limited life expectancy and minimal chance of improvement with surgery are also a contraindication.[1]

Cardiac assessment should be performed according to the American Heart Association guidelines, last published in 2007 with a focused update in 2009.[3,6] These latest guidelines indicate that very few patients require preoperative cardiac testing, such as those with unstable coronary syndromes, decompensated heart failure, severe valvular disease, or atrial or ventricular arrhythmias. This is because recent evidence shows that perioperative revascularization is not helpful and may be more harmful for most patients with asymptomatic disease.[6]

There are difficulties, however, in assessing bariatric patients. To use reliable clinical predictors and consider the patients to be asymptomatic, the patients have to be able to perform activities that require at least 4 metabolic equivalents.[3] These activities include doing housework, climbing a flight of stairs, or walking up a hill. Many bariatric patients are unable to do this because of multiple factors, including osteoarthritis, lower extremity edema and wounds, prolonged immobility, or real cardiopulmonary disease. These factors make the assessment of bariatric patients difficult. Moreover, the actual cardiac testing modalities also can be limited because exercise stress

Table 1
Preoperative tests ordered in bariatric patients at initial evaluation

Laboratory Tests	Radiology/Other
Complete blood counts	Ultrasonography (all except those with prior cholecystectomy)
Electrolyte level, BUN/Cr, liver function tests	Electrocardiogram for those older than 40 years or younger if indicated
Hemoglobin A1c level, glucose level	Sleep study and referral when indicated
Iron level, total iron binding capacity	Cardiac testing selectively
Vitamin B12, folate, thiamine, vitamin D, and calcium levels and lipid panel	Upper GI study and/or endoscopy

It is important to elicit any underlying renal disease, liver dysfunction (eg, nonalcoholic steatohepatitis), diabetes, and nutritional deficiencies. Abnormalities in these tests rarely disqualify patients from bariatric surgery and are more for optimizing their health status to reduce perioperative complications.

Abbreviation: BUN/Cr, blood urea nitrogen to creatinine ratio.

testing may not be possible because of the factors already mentioned. The accuracy of nuclear testing, such as thallium scanning, can be diminished in patients with a BMI less than 30.[3] Transthoracic echocardiography can reveal poor images. Some investigators believe that transesophageal dobutamine stress echocardiography may be more reliable than other tests, but it is more invasive and expensive.[3] The other important factor that is tied in with pulmonary testing and can increase perioperative risk is significant pulmonary hypertension caused by chronic obesity–related hypoventilation and sleep apnea. It is important to screen for this hypertension as well. Because of these difficulties, there is a low threshold to screen asymptomatic patients who have intermediate cardiac risk factors or a combination of risks such as prior myocardial infarction or known coronary artery disease (CAD), compensated congestive heart failure, renal insufficiency, advanced age and diabetes, smoking, and/or a strong family history of CAD.

The prevalence of obstructive sleep apnea (OSA) is 39% to 71% in bariatric patients.[3,7] Many patients are unaware that they have OSA until they come for a bariatric evaluation. Initial screening is done with a history taking and physical examination and a daytime sleepiness evaluation, such as the Epworth sleepiness scale, but most patients are referred for a polysomnography or sleep study. Up to 82% of those who are referred for a sleep study are diagnosed with sleep apnea.[3] It is important to initiate continuous positive airway pressure (CPAP) or bilevel positive airway pressure (BiPAP) before surgery to ensure a good fitting mask and patient compliance. Use of CPAP or BiPAP perioperatively, such as in the recovery room after surgery, and during sleep periods, day or night, postoperatively is very important to reduce hypoxemia, hypercarbia, and significant pulmonary vasoconstriction. The use of these devices are extremely important in patients with preexisting pulmonary hypertension because these patients can have respiratory failure, acute right heart failure, and cardiovascular collapse due to hypoventilation.

Limited data exist for the recommendation of routine screening for *Helicobacter pylori* in bariatric patients. The rate of *H pylori* positivity in bariatric patients is similar to that in the normal population and varies from 10% to 37.5%.[8–12] *H pylori* infection was not necessarily associated with symptomatic patients. The importance of this finding lies in the fact that some retrospective studies have shown a positive correlation between *H pylori* infection and the rate of postoperative marginal ulceration after Roux-en-Y gastric bypass (RYGB).[9,13] However, with other methods of testing for *H pylori* infection (serum titer, breath test), endoscopy may not be required to check for positivity.

ENDOSCOPIC EVALUATION

The role of routine endoscopy for preoperative evaluation in bariatric patients is controversial. The main question in the current cost sensitive health care environment is whether routine endoscopy will alter management. To answer this question, it should be know what the rate of abnormal findings is when routine endoscopy is performed and if these findings will change the operation. Abnormal findings on preoperative endoscopy in bariatric patients have been reported to be from 10% to 90%.[8] This great variability is likely because it is unknown whether all patients undergoing surgery underwent endoscopy or if symptomatic patients only were screened.[8] The rate of hiatal hernias reported in the literature in bariatric patients is 0.54% in the largest series[9] and 40%, 63%, and 90% in 3 other series.[8] It is thus difficult to make any sort of concrete judgment based on the available literature. However, clinically significant findings such as significant erosive esophagitis/gastritis, active ulcer disease, and Barrett syndrome have been reported in 12% of patients.[8] Moreover, significant lesions requiring change in surgical plans, such as those in gastric or esophageal cancer, or gastrointestinal stromal tumors (GISTs)/carcinoids have been found in 0.16% to 0.70% of patients.[8] However, hiatal hernias, according to some surgeons, can be recognized intraoperatively and repaired at the time without necessarily requiring a preoperative endoscopy. The yield of endoscopy is much higher in symptomatic patients, and we perform an endoscopy preoperatively in all symptomatic patients. In addition, in all patients with a gastric band, an esophagram is performed preoperatively to assess for a hiatal hernia and to get a general measure of esophageal motility.

If endoscopy is performed in preoperative bariatric patients, the findings can be grouped into 4 categories to aid in management: group I, normal or findings that do not affect medical or surgical management; group II, findings that require some medical therapy and may delay surgery but do not affect surgical management; group III, findings that may change surgical management; and group IV, findings that are absolute contraindications to surgery. We use this method to describe the findings and utility of preoperative endoscopy.

Group I: Normal or Findings Not Affecting Medical or Surgical Management

The prevalence of normal endoscopy has already been discussed. Findings not affecting management include some benign/hyperplastic gastric or duodenal polyps, esophageal webs, mild/grade A esophagitis, and small hiatal hernias in patients undergoing RYGB. The incidence of nonneoplastic polyps in the duodenum and stomach has been reported to be 1.3% to 3.0%.[10,14,15] The lesions are biopsied and are potentially more relevant in patients loosing access to them, such as those undergoing gastric bypass as opposed to those having a band or undergoing sleeve gastrectomy. These lesions, however, do not usually change surgical management because of their benign nature and lack of progression to a malignancy. Mild esophagitis/gastritis is not very concerning, and the role of *H pylori* has been discussed already.

Group II: Findings Requiring Medical Management and Delay But Not Change in Surgical Management

Esophagitis and gastritis have been reported in around a third of the patients, with more severe esophagitis found in patients with a BMI more than 40.[7,11,12] Theoretically, making an anastomosis or a staple line across inflamed tissue may worsen outcomes, and certain procedures, such as the adjustable gastric band surgery and sleeve gastrectomy, may worsen reflux symptoms initially. So it makes sense to medically treat the inflammation, including *H pylori* eradication if indicated, before surgery. Whether a repeat endoscopy is needed is questionable, but antacid therapy should be continued perioperatively.

Gastric and duodenal ulcers are found in 1% to 3% of endoscopies.[8–11,14] These ulcers have been found in around 1% of asymptomatic patients as well.[16] These ulcers should be biopsied and aggressively treated. We recommend a repeat endoscopy to document healing, especially if a gastric bypass is planned and access would be lost to the remnant stomach and duodenum. It is also be best to avoid an anastomosis or staple line at the site of a gastric ulcer, and perioperative stress can potentially worsen active ulcer disease. Other findings, such as food bezoars, may prompt a gastroparesis or further psychological workup and may or may not alter surgical plans.

Group III: Findings That May Delay Surgery and May Affect/Change Surgical Management

Barrett mucosa has been reported in less than 1% to 5% or higher in preoperative endoscopies.[9,17,18] Barrett mucosa delays management in that biopsy results have to be analyzed. Because access to the esophagus is maintained in all bariatric surgeries and gastric bypass is a good antireflux operation, if no dysplasia is found, then usually one can proceed to surgery and continue postoperative surveillance. Other options, such as local ablative therapy, are still feasible in these patients. In fact, because Barrett esophagus is thought to be caused by chronic acid and/or bile reflux, gastric bypass may be a better option for morbidly obese patients with reflux rather than a sleeve gastrectomy, laparoscopic adjustable gastric band (LAGB) surgery, or fundoplication.

Hiatal hernias should be repaired because they can cause symptoms postoperatively, especially dysphagia if the pouch and gastrojejunostomy/anastomosis is allowed to slide above the hiatus. Although this repair may be favorable for preoperative endoscopy, it is debatable because hiatal hernias can be recognized and treated intraoperatively. Although smaller hiatal hernias may be less consequential in a gastric bypass, they are very important in LAGB. Large hiatal hernias can be considered a contraindication for LAGB. Common complications of LAGB are pouch dilation and slips/gastric prolapse. Parikh and colleagues[19] found that 27% of slips and 53% of pouch dilations were associated with hiatal hernia at the time of reoperation. Gulkarov and colleagues[20] recently published a report on a large series of 1298 patients undergoing an LAGB and 520 patients undergoing LAGB and hiatal hernia repair. The rate of reoperation for band slip or pouch dilation was 5.6% in the LAGB group and 1.7% in the group with concomitant hiatal hernia repair. The investigators believe that as the patients loose weight and loose some of their abundant visceral/epiphrenic fat, the crural defect becomes larger, increasing the size of the hiatal hernia and contributing to more slips. Some of these hiatal hernias are not diagnosed by endoscopy or an upper gastrointestinal (GI) contrast study but by intraoperatively looking at the hiatus, especially after clearing the gastroesophageal fat pad. It seems to be important to know whether there is a hiatal hernia or not, and although endoscopy is a good method to look for hiatal hernias, it is by no means foolproof.

Finding gastric polyps can alter surgical plans. Finding a few fundic gland polyps in patients on chronic proton pump inhibitor may not change management. Finding multiple large polyps requires multiple biopsies. If dysplasia, adenomatous polyps, or any other reason for which surveillance is needed is found, then either an operation that maintains endoscopic access, such as the LAGB surgery or sleeve gastrectomy, or a resectional gastric bypass through which the stomach remnant is resected is warranted. Similar principles apply to duodenal polyps except that resection is not a feasible option, so surveillance must be maintained. These principles also apply to carcinoids and GISTs. GISTs have been found in around 0.7% of bariatric patients, and depending on their anatomic location, GISTs usually can be resected and the bariatric procedure still done.[8]

Group IV: Contraindication to Bariatric Surgery

Barrett esophagus with high-grade dysplasia is considered a relative contraindication to bariatric surgery. Because esophageal cancer and an esophagectomy are distinct possibilities, it is best to preserve the gastric conduit and avoid any dissection around the hiatus. As some of the local therapies develop and advance and as more data become available about its safety, especially oncological safety, then a gastric bypass (a good antireflux operation) may become an option after initial local therapy.

The finding of any malignancy, such as esophageal, gastric, duodenal, or pancreatic malignancy, in the upper GI system is considered a contraindication to bariatric surgery. This finding is rare in patients being considered for bariatric surgery and has been reported in less than 0.2% of patients in the various series published about preoperative endoscopy in bariatric patients.[8,14]

Varices, portal hypertension, and advanced cirrhosis are a contraindication to surgery. These conditions can cause significant intraoperative and postoperative bleeding as well as decompensation of liver disease. Although there are reports of patients with grade 1 esophageal varices who after undergoing a preoperative liver biopsy and evaluation underwent a RYGB successfully, this procedure is not routine.[16]

GUIDELINES

The need for routine preoperative endoscopy in all patients may be controversial; however, the specialty societies have guidelines. This section is a synopsis of the guidelines.

The guidelines from the European Association for Endoscopic Surgery recommend preoperative endoscopy in all bariatric patients regardless of symptoms. This preoperative endoscopy may be substituted with an upper GI barium study, but a preoperative evaluation is necessary in all patients.[21]

The Standards of Practice Committee of the American Society for Gastrointestinal Endoscopy (ASGE) published guidelines in 2008. These guidelines are also endorsed by the Society of American Gastrointestinal and Endoscopic Surgeons.[22]

- An esophagogastroduodenoscopy (EGD) should be performed in all patients with upper GI tract symptoms if they are to undergo bariatric surgery. (Grade 2C)
- An EGD is to be considered in all patients undergoing a RYGB, even if asymptomatic. (Grade 3)
- In asymptomatic patients not undergoing an endoscopy, noninvasive *H pylori* testing is recommended, followed by treatment if the results are positive. (Grade 3)
- In asymptomatic patients being considered for adjustable gastric banding, upper endoscopy should be considered to look for large hiatal hernias that may alter surgical management. (Grade 2C).

Grade 2C recommendation is based on observational studies with some unclear benefit and Grade 3 recommendations are expert opinion only. For details see the *User's Guide to the Medical Literature*.[23]

The American Society of Metabolic and Bariatric Surgery (ASMBS) published broad bariatric surgery guidelines trying to address all aspects. There is no strong recommendation for upper endoscopy. The ASMBS recommends performing upper endoscopy in symptomatic patients and considering upper endoscopy in asymptomatic patients.[24] There are no data that recommend performing routine endoscopy on all patients being considered for bariatric surgery. However, most experts recommend routine preoperative endoscopy in all symptomatic patients and a low threshold in the asymptomatic patient. We perform routine preoperative endoscopy in all symptomatic patients. For asymptomatic patients undergoing an LAGB, an esophagram/upper GI series with barium or an upper endoscopy is done. The threshold for preoperative testing also depends on resources available to a health system and the prevalence of significant upper GI pathologic condition in particular geographic locations around the world.

POSTOPERATIVE MANAGEMENT

Postoperative care involves monitoring standard problems such as bleeding and also issues particular to morbidly obese patients. Patients with sleep apnea should be encouraged to bring their own CPAP masks because these masks are usually the best fit. Some patients with significant pulmonary hypertension and sleep apnea can be placed on CPAP right after extubation. Others can be started that night and should have it on during all sleep periods. There is not much evidence that suggest that starting earlier on CPAP puts fresh upper GI anastomosis at risk.[1] Like in all abdominal surgeries, pulmonary toilet, incentive spirometry, head of bed elevation, and early ambulation are all very beneficial. All bariatric floors should have lift teams or enough trained personnel or mechanical aids to safely get morbidly obese people up and to ambulate very early on.

Morbidly obese patients intuitively seem to be at high risk for venous thromboembolism (VTE). However, some studies have shown that the rate of deep vein thrombosis (DVT) is around 2.5%.[1] This rate is lower than the DVT rate of a broad general surgery population, but that may be because there are no patients with cancer and no patients with emergency surgery in this group. This lower rate is also because most bariatric surgeons administer DVT prophylaxis, even preoperatively. Pneumatic compression devices are placed before anesthesia induction, and early ambulation is a must. There is no consensus or guideline statement regarding what dose or frequency to administer pharmacologic prophylaxis. Pharmacologically, it makes sense to administer higher doses to morbidly obese people. Low-molecular weight heparin and unfractionated heparin have not been compared with each other specifically in the bariatric population, but when anti-Xa levels have been followed for these patients, 30 mg twice daily dosing of enoxaparin has been found to be inadequate in most patients and even 40 mg twice daily may be barely adequate in about half the patients, especially in those with a higher BMI.[25] We give 40 mg subcutaneously preoperatively and continue 40 mg twice daily until discharge. In patients with a BMI more than 55 to 60, we may increase the enoxaparin to 60 mg twice daily or follow anti-Xa levels. Continuing pharmacologic prophylaxis for around 2 weeks after discharge is often recommended for these patients with high BMI; however, the practice is variable and there are no standard recommendations. A recent retrospective study looked at extended prophylaxis for 1 to 3 weeks postoperatively and reported a rate of 0% of VTE in 735 patients.[26] Prophylactic vena cava filters are reserved for very high-risk patients (multiple prior VTEs, significant pulmonary hypertension) who cannot receive pharmacologic prophylaxis, and the retrievable versions are preferred.

Oral intake is resumed rather quickly after bariatric surgery, unlike in typical upper GI surgery. Bariatric clear liquids (low or no sugar, noncarbonated) are started on postoperative day 1. Some physicians get an upper GI examination on postoperative day 1 to rule out a leak or obstruction, but this practice is variable and evidence is scant. Patients are encouraged to consume 1 to 2 ounces of fluid every hour initially, and by postoperative day 2, patients can drink ad lib and are encouraged to take in around 64 ounces per 2 L of fluid a day. At home, patients advance their diet weekly through several phases. In the second week, patients advance to full liquids, then to pureed food, and then soft food, and by 1 month they advance to a more regular low-fat, low/no-sugar diet. It is very important to supplement the intake initially with protein drinks that are appropriate for the phase of diet. At this point, patients who still have their gallbladder but no stones are placed on ursodiol for the first 6 months to decrease the chance of stone formation with the rapid weight loss.

Table 2
Nutritional supplements recommended postbariatric surgery (from a Cleveland Clinic patient handout)

Mandatory	Dosage Per Day	Suggested Schedule
Adult multivitamin and mineral	1–2[a]	AM
Vitamin B12	500 mg	AM
Iron	27–28 mg	PM with vitamin C
Vitamin C	500 mg	PM with iron
Calcium citrate with vitamin D	1200–1500 mg	Take with meals in divided doses
Optional		
Zinc	10–20 mg	AM
Stool softener	As directed	Take with iron dose

[a] Adult.
Abbreviations: AM, morning; PM, evening.

Bariatric surgery patients can have nutrient deficiencies to start with that can be exacerbated postoperatively. It is very important for these patients to take micronutrient supplements. Micronutrient and macronutrient deficiencies may occur post gastric bypass, with the most common ones listed in **Table 2**. Our patients follow the supplemental guidelines shown in **Table 2**. In addition to information about what to eat, it is important to counsel bariatric patients on how to eat. Apart from extensive sessions with the dieticians/nutritionists and regular reinforcement, patients receive specific handouts (**Box 1**) to help reinforce the change in eating habits.

Box 1
Nutrition tips after bariatric surgery given to patients (from a Cleveland Clinic patient handout)

1. Protein as the number 1 food. Always eat lean protein food first to meet the 60 g of lean protein intake a day. Lean protein can be 28 g of meat (chicken, turkey, fish, beef, or pork), 28 g of low-fat cheese, 2 tablespoons peanut butter, 1 egg, and quarter cup of low-fat cottage cheese.
2. No skipping meals. Eat at least 3 meals a day. Having 1 to 2 small high-protein snacks may be beneficial if a gap of more than 4 hours is taken in between meals. Small frequent meals help to prevent filling up of the pouch too fast and to keep the metabolism burning.
3. Eat at the table. Use a plate or dish and sit down. Take 30 minutes to eat meals. Avoid eating at the counter or cupboards, in front of the refrigerator, in other areas of the home, or in front of the television or computer.
4. Portion control. Serve smaller portions. Cut up chicken in smaller pieces. Use a salad plate as the dinner plate or baby spoons to prevent overeating. Slow down with eating, chew foods thoroughly, and stop when feeling full. Keep serving dishes off the table.
5. Liquids 101. Drinking 6 to 8 cups of caffeine-free, calorie-free, and noncarbonated beverages a day is a must. Do not drink with meals; stop drinking 30 minutes before the meal, eat, and then wait 30 minutes after the meal to drink again. This will prevent nausea and vomiting. Sip on fluids in between meals.
6. Take your vitamin/mineral supplements daily. Take multivitamin and calcium supplements daily according to the doctor's prescription. Additional vitamin B12, vitamin C, and iron may be required.
7. Your new way of life. Try not to think of this weight loss surgery as a diet but as a new way of life not only for oneself but also for one's family and friends. These healthy habits are a lifestyle change for now and forever.

Table 3
Follow-up plan for postbariatric surgery (from a Cleveland Clinic patient handout)

	1 wk	1 mo	3 mo	6 mo	9 mo	1 y	Annually
Surgical Follow-up	✓	✓	✓	✓	✓	✓	✓
Laboratory Work	—	—	—	✓	—	✓	✓
Dietary Counseling	—	✓	✓	As needed	—	—	—
Psychological Counseling	—	✓	As needed	—	—	—	—
Exercise Prescription	—	✓	As needed	—	—	—	—

FOLLOW-UP

Follow-up after bariatric surgery, like the preoperative period, is more involved than that for most surgical procedures. Our general follow-up plan is shown in **Table 3**. In addition to following up with the surgeon at the intervals shown, the patients can schedule shared medical appointments. These are group sessions with up to 12 bariatric patients who are led by the medical physician trained in bariatric medicine (bariatrician). These sessions last for 90 minutes and include individual monitoring of diet progression, medications, nutritional supplements, exercise, blood work, and disease management. In addition, patients have the opportunity to talk with each other about their own experience and/or concerns. This appointment schedule is somewhat modified for patients with gastric band depending on whether the surgeon does the band adjustments. We do our own band adjustments so we see our band patients every 2 months for the first year and every 3 months for the second year for follow-up and a band adjustment under fluoroscopy. We see them annually thereafter if all is well. The laboratories that we check annually are the same as those that are checked preoperatively, and are listed in **Table 1**. Any abnormalities in follow-up, such as dysphagia, nausea, or epigastric pain, in the short term and failure of weight loss, weight regain, malnutrition, or anemia in the long term, elicit further investigations and more rigorous follow-up.

SUMMARY

The preoperative evaluation and postoperative follow-up of the bariatric patient is a true multidisciplinary team effort. Patients can have significant undiagnosed metabolic diseases when first seen that can pose a significant challenge in the perioperative period. Preoperative preparation of the patient not only from a medical standpoint but also from the psychological and behavioral modification standpoint is extremely important. The patient must proceed through the course of evaluation as well informed as possible. The patients have to understand that bariatric surgery is a lifelong commitment and that this surgery should be reinforced with frequent postoperative follow-up and monitoring.

REFERENCES

1. Schauer PR, Schirmer DB, Brethauer SA. Patient selection, preoperative assessment, and preparation. In: Schauer PR, Schirmer DB, Brethauer SA, editors. Minimally invasive bariatric surgery. Springer; 2007. p. 57–64. Chapter 8.
2. Gastrointestinal surgery for severe obesity. National Institutes of Health Consensus Development Conference Statement. Am J Clin Nutr 1992;55:615s–9s.
3. Kuruba R, Koche LS, Murr MM. Preoperative assessment and perioperative care of patients undergoing bariatric surgery. Med Clin North Am 2007;91:339–51.

4. Liu RC, Sabnis AA, Forsyth C, et al. The effects of acute preoperative weight loss on laparoscopic Roux-en-Y gastric bypass. Obes Surg 2005;15(10):1396–402.
5. Flancbaum L, Drake V, Colarusso T, et al. Initial experience with bariatric surgery in asymptomatic human immunodeficiency virus-infected patients. Surg Obes Relat Dis 2005;1(2):P73–6.
6. Fleisher LA, Beckman JA, Brown KA, et al. ACC/AHA 2007 Guidelines on perioperative cardiovascular evaluation and care for noncardiac surgery. Circulation 2007;116:e418–500.
7. Frey WC, Pilcher J. Obstructive sleep-related breathing disorders in patients evaluated for bariatric surgery. Obes Surg 2003;13:676–83.
8. Mong C, Van Dam J, Morton J, et al. Preoperative endoscopic screening for laparoscopic Roux-en-Y gastric bypass has a low yield for anatomic findings. Obes Surg 2008;18:1067–73.
9. Schirmer B, Erenoglu C, Miller A. Flexible endoscopy in the management of patients undergoing Roux-en-Y gastric bypass. Obes Surg 2002;12:634–8.
10. Loewen M, Giovanni J, Barba C. Screening endoscopy before bariatric surgery: a series of 448 patients. Surg Obes Relat Dis 2008;4:709–14.
11. Korenkov M, Sauerland S, Shah S, et al. Is routine preoperative upper endoscopy in gastric banding patients really necessary? Obes Surg 2006;16:45–7.
12. Almeida AM, Cotrim HP, Santos AS, et al. Preoperative upper gastrointestinal endoscopy in obese patients undergoing bariatric surgery: is it necessary? Surg Obes Relat Dis 2008;4:144–51.
13. Papasavas PK, Gagne DJ, Donnelly PE, et al. Prevalence of *Helicobacter pylori* infection and value of preoperative testing and treatment in patients undergoing laparoscopic Roux-en-Y gastric bypass. Surg Obes Relat Dis 2008;4:383–8.
14. Munoz R, Ibanez L, Salinas J, et al. Importance of routine preoperative upper GI endoscopy: why all patients should be evaluated? Obes Surg 2009;19:427–31.
15. Madan AK, Speck KE, Hiler ML. Routine preoperative upper endoscopy for laparoscopic gastric bypass: is it necessary? Am Surg 2004;70:684–6.
16. Azagury D, Dumonceau JM, Morel P, et al. Preoperative work-up in asymptomatic patients undergoing Roux en-Y gastric bypass: is endoscopy mandatory? Obes Surg 2006;16:1304–11.
17. Csendes A, Burgos AM, Smok G, et al. Endoscopic and histologic findings of the foregut in 426 patients with morbid obesity. Obes Surg 2007;17:28–34.
18. Sharaf RN, Weinshel EH, Bini EJ, et al. Endoscopy plays an important preoperative role in bariatric surgery. Obes Surg 2004;14:1367–72.
19. Parikh MS, Fielding GA, Ren CJ. U.S. experience with 749 laparoscopic adjustable gastric bands: intermediate outcomes. Surg Endosc 2005;19:1631–5.
20. Gulkarov I, Wetterau M, Ren CJ, et al. Hiatal hernia repair at the initial laparoscopic adjustable gastric band operation reduces the need for reoperation. Surg Endosc 2008;22:1035–41.
21. Sauerland S, Angrisani L, Belachew M, et al, European Association for Endoscopic Surgery. Obesity surgery: evidence-based guidelines of the European Association for Endoscopic Surgery (EAES). Surg Endosc 2005;19:200–21.
22. ASGE Standards of Practice Committee, Anderson MA, Gan SI, et al. Role of endoscopy in the bariatric surgery patient. Gastrointest Endosc 2008;68(1):1–10.
23. Guyatt G, Sinclair J, Cook D, et al. Moving from evidence to action. Grading recommendations: a qualitative approach. In: Guyatt G, Rennie D, editors. Users' guides to the medical literature. Chicago: AMA Press; 2002. p. 599–608.

24. Mechanick JI, Kushner RF, Sugerman HJ, et al. American Association of Clinical Endocrinologists, The Obesity Society, and American Society for Metabolic & Bariatric Surgery Medical guidelines for clinical practice for the perioperative nutritional, metabolic, and nonsurgical support of the bariatric surgery patient. Surg Obes Relat Dis 2008;4:S109–84.
25. Rowan BO, Kul DA, Lee MD, et al. Anti-Xa levels in bariatric surgery patients receiving prophylactic enoxaparin. Obes Surg 2008;18(2):162–6.
26. Magee CJ, Barry J, Javed S, et al. Extended thromboprophylaxis reduces incidence of postoperative venous thromboembolism in laparoscopic bariatric surgery. Surg Obes Relat Dis 2010;6(3):322–5.

Medical Management of Postsurgical Complications: The Bariatric Surgeon's Perspective

Michael J. Lee, MD, Daniel J. Scott, MD*

KEYWORDS

- Bariatric • Complications • Restrictive
- Malabsorptive • Combined

The prevalence of morbid obesity continues to increase at an alarming pace. Related comorbidities such as diabetes, hypertension, hyperlipidemia, and cardiovascular disease are responsible for 2.5 million deaths per year according to the World Health Organization.[1] The approximate loss of life for each morbidly obese individual is 12 years compared with nonobese persons.[2] Obesity is considered a disease of genetic predisposition and maladjusted behavior; however its cause is multifactorial and not yet completely understood. Perhaps because of ignorance and social stigmatization, morbid obesity is not yet fully accepted as a disease by the public or even among physicians. Complications resulting from obesity-related surgery may not be well received by the public and bariatric surgery is closely scrutinized in some environments.

A BRIEF HISTORY

A thorough insight in clinical outcomes and managing complications first requires an understanding of procedures from a historical perspective. Through clinical observation, surgeons have learned that the shortened gut leads to massive weight loss. Early in the 1950s, it was observed that short gut syndrome could be manipulated to advantage by creating a malabsorptive procedure to provide massive weight loss and weight maintenance.

The first purposeful bariatric operation manifested as the jejunoileal bypass. By limiting intestinal length and surface area, malabsorption of ingested food leads to decreased body mass and also reduces the caloric need to accommodate the

Department of Surgery, Southwestern Center for Minimally Invasive Surgery, University of Texas Southwestern Medical Center, 5323 Harry Hines Boulevard, Dallas, TX 75390-9156, USA
* Corresponding author.
E-mail address: daniel.scott@utsouthwestern.edu

Gastrointest Endoscopy Clin N Am 21 (2011) 241–256
doi:10.1016/j.giec.2011.02.012 giendo.theclinics.com
1052-5157/11/$ – see front matter

decreased body mass, achieving a metabolic equilibrium. The jejunoileal bypass was effective in malabsorption resulting in massive weight loss but carried many side effects, such as gas-bloating, steatorrhea, electrolyte disturbances, nephrolithiasis, and hepatic fibrosis, and was therefore later abandoned. In the 1960s and 1970s, malabsorptive procedures combined with restrictive procedures, such as the Roux-en-Y gastric bypass (RYGB), biliopancreatic diversion, and duodenal switch, gained popularity. In the 1980s, gastroplasties in various forms, such as stapling and banding, came into favor. Now, favorable outcomes support laparoscopic sleeve gastrectomy as an attractive option.[3,4]

Trial and error with malabsorptive, restrictive, and combined procedures, along with minimal access techniques, have progressed bariatric surgery into its contemporary form. In the laparoscopic era, the RYGB, adjustable gastric band, and sleeve gastrectomy are favored bariatric operations because of their efficacy and acceptable complication rates. There is no single bariatric operation suitable to all patients. Ultimately, multiple facets should be carefully examined to balance lifestyle and risk tolerance for complications.

COMPARISONS

Morbid obesity continues to occur at an epidemic rate. Fewer than 40,000 annual bariatric cases were reported before the advent of the laparoscopic era.[4] That number is projected to increase to more than 200,000 annually.[5] Although complication rates are among the lowest reported for major abdominal procedures, bariatric surgery remains in high profile and complications are not well received by the public, patients, or medical community.

In the largest review and meta-analysis of more than 85,000 patients, mortalities for bariatric procedures were among the lowest reported in the global surgical community (**Table 1**). Reported outcomes revealed a total 30 day mortality of 0.28% and a 2-year mortality of 0.35% for all bariatric procedures.[5] Mortality between open and laparoscopic operations for all procedures similarly remained low. Men had a disproportionately high 30-day mortality compared with women, 4.74:0.13, consistent with technical challenges as well as medical problems associated with android fat distribution. The superobese with body mass indices (BMIs) equal to or greater than 50 had a higher 30-day mortality (1.25%), and the elderly (>65 years) had a 30-day mortality of 0.34%.[5]

In comparison between open and laparoscopic operations, a randomized trial by Nguyen and colleagues[6] of 155 patients discovered no difference in mortality between patients having laparoscopic versus open gastric bypass. However, patients having

Table 1
Bariatric mortality

	≤30 d Mortality (%)	>30 d to 2 y Mortality (%)
Total	0.28	0.35
Restrictive	0.30 open 0.07 laparoscopic	0.22 open 0.01 laparoscopic
Combined	0.41 open 0.16 laparoscopic	0.69 open 0.09 laparoscopic
Malabsorptive	0.76 open 1.11 laparoscopic	0.85 open N/A laparoscopic

Data from Buchwald H, Estok R, Fahrbach K, et al. Trends in mortality in bariatric surgery: a systematic review and meta-analysis. Surgery 2007;142:629.

laparoscopic gastric bypass had a lower incidence of infectious complications, lower incidence of incisional hernias, less operative blood loss, shorter hospital stay, reduced frequency of late anastomotic stricture, and earlier return to work and activities of daily living.

Other studies, including large case series, support similar complication rates. In a review by Parikh and colleagues[7] of 780 laparoscopic bariatric operations, including LAP-BAND, laparoscopic RYGB (LRYGB), and biliopancreatic diversion bypass with or without duodenal switch (BPD ± DS), there was 1 reported late death. Major complications, including organ resection, irreversible deficits, and death, occurred in 0.2% for the LAP-BAND, 2% LRYGB, and 5% BPD ± DS.

Early initial results were not as uniform. Early data from Flum and colleagues[8] revealed that mortality among Medicare patients 65 years and older was significantly higher than for patients younger than 65 years at 1 year, 11.1% compared with 3.9%. Men also had a higher 1-year mortality: 7.5% compared with 3.7% in women. In contrast, Hallowell and colleagues[9] found no difference in mortality in their series of 928 Medicare patients, and argued that that there is inevitable selection bias. They attribute their results to careful patient selection, intensive preoperative education, and expert management.

Pregnancy and fertility following bariatric surgery has shown favorable outcome to those who undergo initial bariatric surgery then pursue pregnancy.[10] Although, at first, the potential for neural tube defects from folate and nutrient deficiency following bariatric surgery must be considered, data support lower adverse maternal and neonatal outcomes in women who become pregnant after having had bariatric surgery compared with rates in pregnant women who are obese.[10] Most advocate waiting at least 1 year after bariatric surgery, until a nutritional and metabolic steady state is reached, before pregnancy.[10,11] Close coordination of care between gynecologists and surgeons is paramount to ensure that nutrition and potential complications are monitored in this population.

Bariatric surgery in the adolescent population remains controversial. Proponents favor early intervention to prevent chronic morbidities, whereas opponents argue that adolescents do not exhaust behavioral and medical options. Long-term data are still lacking, but bariatric surgery in adolescents seems to be as well tolerated as in adults when performed in high-volume centers of excellence.[12,13]

Most series show that bariatric surgery can be performed with low rates of perioperative mortality. Overall, the mortality is extremely low compared with rates for other major operations such as aortic aneurysm repair (3.9%), coronary artery bypass graft (3.5%), esophagectomy (9.9%), pancreatectomy (8.3%), and pediatric cardiac surgery (5.4%).[5] Societies such as the American Society for Metabolic and Bariatric Surgery (ASMBS), the Society of American Gastrointestinal and Endoscopic Surgeons (SAGES), the Fellowship Council (FC), and the American College of Surgeons (ACS) have taken leadership roles to ensure safety and quality improvement. Like any surgical morbidity and mortality, complications depend on the surgeon's skill, experience, and operative volume, appropriate patient selection, and choice of procedure.

LAP-BAND COMPLICATIONS

The LAP-BAND procedure was approved in 2001 by the US Food and Drug Administration for surgical weight loss (**Table 2**). Considered the least technically difficult among bariatric operations, it is a restrictive procedure with low foreseeable complication rates and potential for reversibility. Early experience with the pars flaccida technique, routine use of postoperative contrast studies, and delayed first band

Table 2
Most common LAP-BAND complications

Complication	Among All Patients (%)
Access port dysfunction	7.3
Gastric pouch dilation ± esophageal dilation	6.6
Band slippage	1.8
Stoma obstruction	1.8
Pneumonia	0.7
Pulmonary embolism	0.4
Trocar site bleeding	0.4

Data from Spivak H, Anwar F, Burton S, et al. The LAP-BAND system in the United States. Surg Endosc 2004;18:200.

adjustments contributed to low complication rates.[14–16] Most series report less than 0.3% mortality.[15,16] Conversion from laparoscopic to open surgery occurs in 1%, most commonly because of extreme hepatomegaly and intraoperative technical difficulty.[15,16] The mean operative time is 40 minutes, mean hospital stay 1 day, and first band adjustments are made at least 3 months after gastric edema subsides.[15] Total LAP-BAND complications may occur up to 35% and 11% may require reoperation.[17] Most complications are minor and manageable in the clinic, and those requiring operations can usually undergo laparoscopic surgery.

Access port (reservoir for adjustments) complications consist of half of all LAP-BAND complications and account for most reoperations.[18] Of all access port complications, port infection is the most frequent. *Staphylococcus aureus* is usually cultured in the wound or from the port itself. Patients may complain of tenderness and have signs of erythema and rubor around the port site. Treatment consists of antibiotics until resolution of infection. Removal of the reservoir, closure of connector tubing, and introduction of the tube into the peritoneal cavity may be necessary. Leaving the port reservoir or connecting tubing within subcutaneous tissue usually fails to adequately treat infection or heal.[18] Esophagoduodenoscopy may also be useful to evaluate the band for erosion, which may also present as an infected port site.

Mechanical or technical problems are the second most common access port complication. Disconnection between the junction of silicone tube and access port occur in 17.7%. Inability to puncture the reservoir and failure to adjust the band occur in 15.6%. Leaking from the tubing outside of the peritoneal cavity occur in 11.1%. Protrusion of the port reservoir through the dermis occurs in 4.45%. Treatment is usually successful in an outpatient setting under local anesthesia by shortening the tube and reconnecting it to the reservoir under fluoroscopy.[14,17,18]

Port site flip can be avoided by using at least 3 nonabsorbable sutures to the fascia to secure a plane and taking care not to injure the tube during subsequent punctures. Using a smaller, flatter port deep under fascia for those who lose a lot of weight and have reservoir protruding in the dermis may become necessary.[18] Also, the surgeon can place the port in the subxiphoid location or left upper quadrant, whichever accommodates less mechanical friction from abdominal wall movement.[14] Alternatively, ports may be fixed using synthetic mesh.[19] In most cases of technical or mechanical port problems outside the peritoneum, minor procedures can be done under local anesthesia without removal of the gastric band itself.

Intra-abdominal complications involving the band present greater challenges in diagnosis and treatment. Upper gastrointestinal (GI) complaints are usually nonspecific and characterized by food intolerance, pain, and feelings of reflux. Dysphagia and vomiting are more ominous signs and warrant careful concern for obstruction. An upper GI contrast study may be valuable in determining band position and gastric configuration. Obtaining additional views in oblique positions may also aid in diagnosis. In addition to the diagnostic difficulty, the discordance of definitions among surgeons adds to the complexity. The terms prolapse, dilation, pouch enlargement, and slippage are variably defined in the literature and warrant clarification. Although most may be treated nonoperatively, several situations are surgical emergencies and require timely and accurate diagnosis.

Pouch enlargement, or concentric dilation refers to the expanded proximal esophageal or gastric lumen resulting from mechanical luminal stretch and compliance (**Fig. 1**). This condition most likely results from patient noncompliance with oral intake instructions, usually from ingesting more than 110-g meals and/or overinflation of the band.[20,21] Patients usually present with nonspecific upper GI complaints without vomiting or dysphagia. If left untreated, dilation may result in a permanent atonic gastric pouch and atonic esophagus in 50%.[17] Unlike band slippage or eccentric prolapse, dilation of the proximal segment is concentric and the band remains in its original 45 degree orientation.[17]

For prevention, most experts make 3 recommendations: (1) reduce gastric pouch to less than 15 cm^3; (2) place gastric-to-gastric sutures to secure the band; (3) position the posterior aspect of the band high and close to the gastroesophageal junction.[14] Early treatment with band deflation, intravenous fluids (IVF) resuscitation, and dietary intake education may reduce symptoms and reverse the effects. If early treatment fails to resolve symptoms, a cause for obstruction should be suspected.

Eccentric prolapse, true prolapse, eccentric dilation, and slippage refer to the condition in which the gastric wall is displaced cranially and the band is displaced caudally.[17] Patients with pouch enlargement or dilation are believed to be predisposed to prolapse.[22] In addition to the upper GI complaints, patients complain of dysphasia and vomiting. A dilated eccentric gastric pouch with displacement of the original configuration of the band are seen on upper GI radiography (UGI) (**Fig. 2**).[17] Various configurations have been described, including anterior versus posterior slippages with differences in band angles; however, this entity in general is considered obstructive and the management is surgical.[23] Because of the larger cross-sectional area at the level of the body compared with the area at the level of the angle of His, complete obstruction is inevitable and this situation is always a surgical emergency.[20]

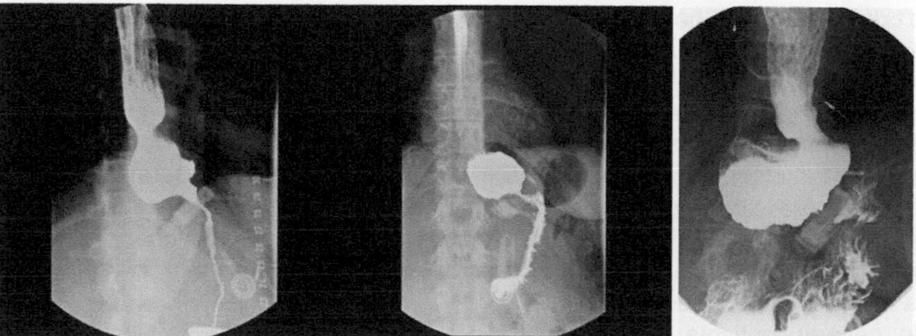

Fig. 1. Symmetric pouch dilation (two left panels) and asymmetrical pouch dilation (right panel).

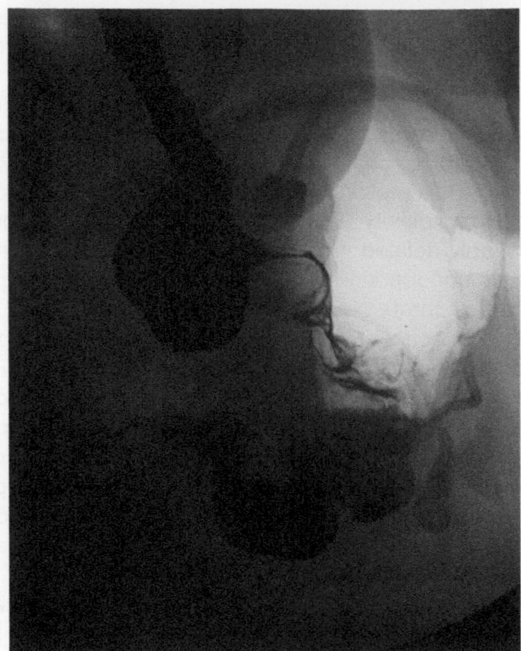

Fig. 2. Band slippage with caudal displacement of the band and partial obstruction of the pouch outlet.

The pars flaccida technique has a lower association with band slippage compared with the earlier perigastric technique.[20,21] Immediate management is similar to that for dilation as described previously. In addition, a nasogastric tube should be inserted to decompress the pouch, enable resolution of edema, and to prevent aspiration. Surgical options include band removal or gastric reduction with band repositioning.[23]

Stoma obstruction refers to the obstruction of food from the gastric pouch to the rest of the stomach. Early postoperative causes are likely from bands applied over a thick gastroesophageal junction (GEJ), incorporating too much tissue inside the band, positioning the band too distally from GEJ, or edema.[14,15] Late postoperative causes may be related to gastric pouch dilation, prolapse, erosion, pouchitis, or esophagitis.[14,15] Patients may present with dysphagia, chest pain, reflux, and vomiting. Patients with early partial obstructions may be managed conservatively with nutritional support, systemic steroids, and diuresis. Most will respond within a few days as the edema subsides; however, patients with complete obstruction, either early or late, may need to undergo exploratory laparoscopy and revisional surgery.

Erosion of the LAP-BAND is rare, occurring in less than 2%.[24] Patients may present with acute peritoneal signs (**Fig. 3**). Most patients present with more chronic or subclinical findings that indicate a port site infection. Chronic erosion may present with port infection. Proposed causes include undetected intraoperative iatrogenic injury and pressure necrosis of the band.[24] Chronic usage of immunosuppressive medications is also believed to greatly increase the risk of erosions. Treatment is surgical for acute presentations. Successful endoscopic retrieval for chronic erosion has also been described.[14,17]

In general, patients receiving a LAP-BAND may present with constellation of symptoms. Decisive clinical judgment is vital to reducing morbidity. Compromise to gastric blood flow is the key concern to avoid gastric necrosis, a rare and devastating

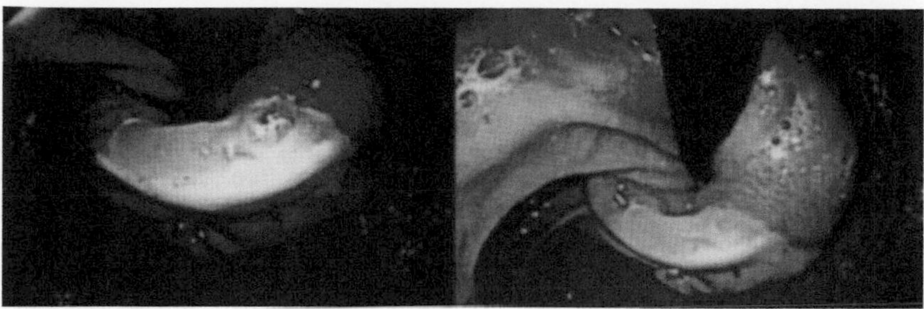

Fig. 3. Band erosion.

consequence of the previously mentioned complications. Basic measures such as IVF resuscitation, NGT decompression, band deflation, and contrasted radiographic imaging are easily forgotten but essential initial maneuvers.

MALABSORPTIVE AND COMBINED PROCEDURE COMPLICATIONS

Among combined restrictive and malabsorptive operations including RYGB, BPD, and DS, total number of complications occurs in 25% (**Table 3**). Severe complications requiring organ resection or lasting disability are less common and occur in 2.3%.[7] These procedures are technically more challenging and require more time and expertise compared with restriction alone with band placement. Mean operative times are 138 minutes for LRYGB and 270 minutes for laparoscopic BPD and DS. Hospital stays vary from 3 to 5 days.[7] The most common bariatric procedure performed in the United States is the RYGB. Variations in limb lengths ultimately determine the severity of malabsorption. The violation of bowel and creation of multiple anastomoses potentiate complications for malabsorptive and combined procedures. Anatomic or structural complications are mostly surgically managed, whereas postgastrectomy syndromes can usually be mitigated medically.

Although uncommon, internal hernia is a serious complication that may present diagnostic challenges. Bariatric surgeons advocate fixation and closure of all potential internal hernia sites to avoid bowel obstruction. Hernia sites may result from

Table 3
Most common bariatric surgical complications

	Complication	Restrictive (%)	Combination (%)
1	Dumping	0.3	14.6
2	Vitamin/mineral deficiency	1.6	11.0
3	Staple line failure	1.5	6.0
4	Infection	3.1	5.3
5	Stenosis/bowel obstruction	2.2	2.7
6	Nausea/vomiting	8.5	2.6
7	Ulceration	1.2	1.2
8	Bleeding	0.5	0.9
9	Splenic injury	0.2	0.8
10	Perioperative death	0.1	0.4

Data from Abell TL, Minocha A. Gastrointestinal complications of bariatric surgery: diagnosis and therapy. Am J Med Sci 2006;331(4):214.

a mesocolic defect, the Petersen defect (space between the Roux limb and the transverse mesocolon), or the jejunal-jejunal window. Internal hernias are reported with an incidence of 1% to 5%.[25–29] More than half of internal hernias result from the mesojejunal mesenteric window.[28] Anecdotal experiences favor the antecolic approach, reducing the number of potential hernia sites from 3 to 2 among some surgeons.[29] Regardless of antecolic or retrocolic configuration, tension-free closure of all potential internal hernia sites with a nonabsorbable running suture has been advocated by most surgeons.[28,29] No randomized controlled trial to date has been conducted examining the 2 approaches. Patients may present with a wide constellation of symptoms and thus internal hernia remains a diagnostic dilemma for physicians. Although not highly specific, recurrent colicky abdominal pain with or without nausea/vomiting is the most common presentation. Most surgeons advocate early diagnostic laparoscopy once internal hernia is suspected because acute intestinal obstruction with necrosis of long segments of bowel cause deleterious consequences.

Postoperative anastomotic leaks are also rare but potentially fatal. Anastomotic leaks occur up to 6%.[26,30–32] Antecolic versus retrocolic Roux limb orientation for more favorable leak rates remains controversial. Most leaks occur at the gastrojejunal anastomosis and rarely at the jejunojejunal anastomosis (**Figs. 4** and **5**).[30–32] Jejunojejunal anastomotic complications are extremely rare and are attributable to poor technique, staple line bleeding, or obstruction.[33] Technical choices include hand-sewn, circular stapled, and linear stapled anastomoses. In addition, the da Vinci robot system has had favorable results using a hand-sewn gastrojejunostomy technique.[34] The goal of an anastomotic repair is to achieve a tension-free, airtight, and well-vascularized anastomosis. Elderly patients, male gender, and patients with

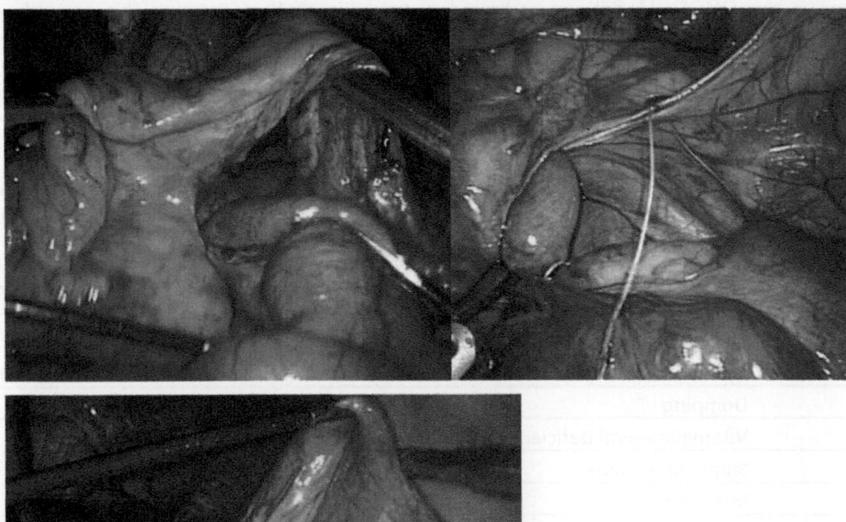

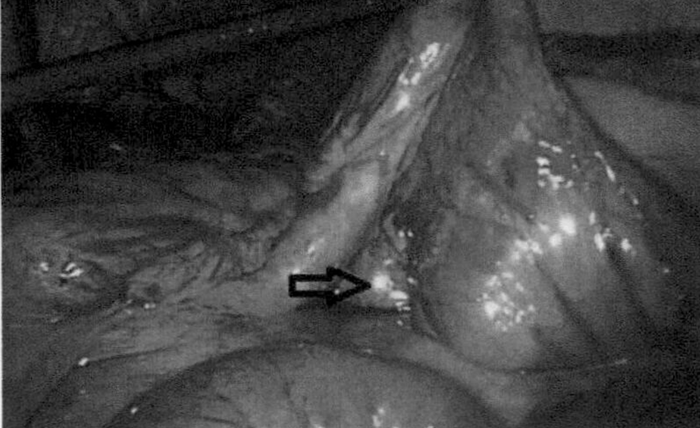

Fig. 4. Clockwise: mesocolic defect, Petersen defect, jejunojejunal defect.

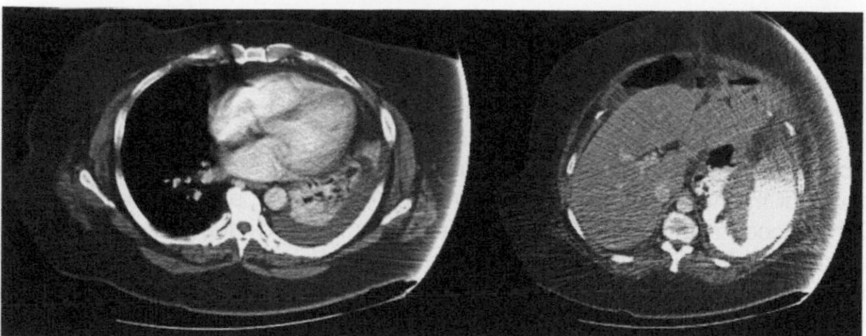

Fig. 5. Gastrojejunostomy leak with left upper quadrant abscess s/p revision RYGB.

higher BMIs are at higher risk for leak.[32] Multifactorial causes include tissue ischemia, tension, and surgeon experience. Patients may present with clinical sepsis including fever, tachycardia, tachypnea, leukocytosis, and shock. UGI may not always detect leaks and a strong clinical suspicion should remain if there are convincing signs because leaks potentiate other major complications such as pulmonary embolism (PE), bowel obstruction, GI bleeding, fistulas, and ventral hernias.

An uncontained leak requires surgery in at least 80% of cases with primary repair and adequate drainage.[26] Extensive inflammation and tissue edema may limit the technical possibility of primary closure and wide drainage may be necessary. Postoperative intensive care unit monitoring, ventilator support, total parenteral nutrition, antibiotics, and deep vein thrombosis (DVT) prophylaxis should also be considered. Small leaks may be asymptomatic and can be managed nonoperatively with percutaneous drainage and antibiotics. Intraoperative leak tests including the use of air or dye may aid in prevention; however, testing and reinforcing suture lines with Lembert suture does not entirely eliminate leaks.

Stenosis usually occurs at the site of an anastomosis. The gastrojejunostomy is the most common site. Poor technique and relative ischemia are contributing factors (**Fig. 6**). Endoscopic balloon dilation has had good therapeutic results and occasionally laparoscopic reoperation is necessary.[25] Stenosis at the mesocolon is less common and usually not technically amenable to endoscopic dilation because of its downstream location and anatomic limitations. Because of the anatomic constraints, this situation, as well as other anatomic complications such as Roux twisting and

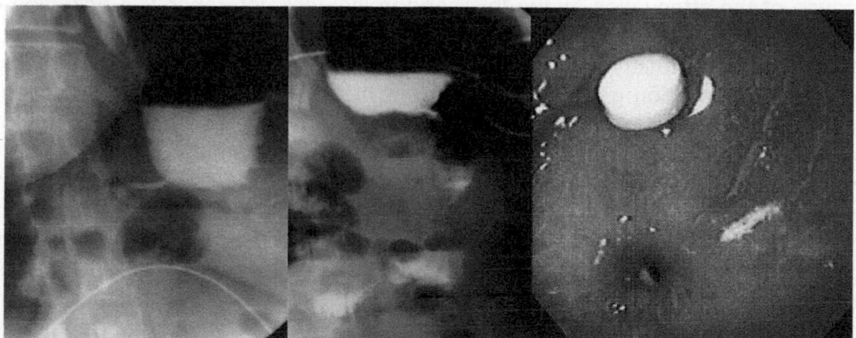

Fig. 6. Gastrojejunostomy stenosis s/p RYGB on UGI (middle and left panels) and esophagogastroduodenoscopy (right panel, note the comparative size of the stoma compared with a tablet).

kinking, are generally managed operatively, although several case studies have shown favorable outcomes for balloon dilation for both gastrojejunal and mesocolic stenosis.[35–37]

Venous thromboembolism and bleeding remain on the opposite spectrum and may complicate bariatric procedures, requiring immediate intervention. Venous thromboembolism remains a difficult clinical diagnosis, especially in the morbidly obese, because of the nonspecificity of symptoms. DVT occurs in up to 4% and PE occurs in 0.2%, accounting for 150,000 deaths annually in the United States.[38] In patients with no prior history of venous thromboembolism, there is a 1% incidence of DVT and preoperative routine screening is not warranted.[38] Venous stasis from prolonged reverse Trendelenburg positioning, decreased venous return during pneumoperitoneum, and muscle paralysis are factors that contribute to the Virchow triad.[39]

Several prophylactic measures, including early ambulation, sequential compression devices, subcutaneous and intravenous unfractionated heparin, and low-molecular-weight heparin have all been tried in various combinations. There are no universally accepted DVT prophylaxis protocols, but most surgeons advocate chemical prophylaxis and sequential pneumatic compression devices throughout preoperative to postoperative period. Subcutaneous unfractionated heparin is favored by most because of its low cost, short half-life, and potential reversibility with protamine if needed. Inferior vena cava filters have been shown to be safe and effective and may benefit those who have a prior history of thromboembolic disease or a contraindication to chemical prophylaxis and those in the superobese range.[40,41] Even with DVT prophylaxis, microscopic evidence of pulmonary emboli can still be found in autopsy studies.[42]

The incidence of early postoperative hemorrhage after open and laparoscopic RYGB ranges between 0.06% and 4.4%. More than half may be intraluminal hematomas causing obstructions.[43] Injury to the spleen should always be considered as a source of bleeding. Bleeding is twice as likely in laparoscopic operations. Advanced age and use of lovenox may increase risk.[43] Differences in BMI, gender, anastomotic technique, and use of postoperative ketorolac have not shown significantly increased bleeding rates. Early recognition of tachycardia, oliguria, and acute hematocrit reduction indicate emergent surgical intervention for hemodynamic instability.

There is a 40% incidence of gallstone formation and up to 14% incidence of symptoms related to cholelithiasis after rapid weight loss.[44–46] Although gallstone disease is highly common, there is no consensus for surgical prophylaxis in morbidly obese patients. Preoperative ultrasound may not be accurate in diagnosing gallstones because of the attenuation by the thick abdominal wall. Intraoperative palpation or ultrasound may be more useful. Proponents for prophylactic cholecystectomy argue that the Y-configuration may limit future endoscopic intervention. Simultaneous cholecystectomy when gallstones are evident has been shown safe and effective. This procedure adds 20 minutes, on average, to the total operative time without increasing hospital stay; however, other groups have documented length of stay to almost double and operative time to increase by up to 1 hour.[44,47] Ursodiol 600 mg daily for 6 months after RYGB for prophylaxis significantly reduces the gallstone formation rate from 32% to 3%.[48] Outside of controlled trials, compliance with this regimen may be poor because of the side effects such as severe nausea, diarrhea, and dry skin/pruritis.[45] Because of the overall low incidence of patients who become symptomatic from gallstones, many surgeons currently do not screen or administer prophylaxis for gallstones.[46]

Postoperative rhabdomyolysis has been described in several case reports with an incidence of 1.4%.[49] Crush injuries, burns, electric shock, and prolonged immobilization may cause rhabdomyolysis through direct muscle injury or muscle ischemia. Strenuous exercise, malignant hyperthermia, myopathies, infections, seizures, and drugs are other potential risk factors. Prolonged anesthesia, lithotomy position, statin therapy, and gluteal decubitus ulceration are specific to the bariatric patient. Preventive measures include using protective padding around buttocks, hips, and shoulders. Intravascular volume depletion may lead to acute renal failure. Once the diagnosis is made, IVF, diuretics, alkalinization of urine, monitoring myoglobin, and creatine kinase levels may help. Late cases may require fasciotomy and surgical debridement.[49–51]

Marginal ulceration is a common complication that may present with upper abdominal pain, progressive food and liquid intolerance, and melena.[26] Risk factors include tissue ischemia, foreign body reaction, tension, medications, and smoking. *Helicobacter pylori* has also been implicated as a risk factor. Upper endoscopy or radiographic imaging is helpful to achieve accurate diagnosis. Antihistamines or proton pump inhibitors and cessation of smoking and ulcerogenic medications are highly effective treatments.[52] In addition, topical agents such as liquid carafate, prostaglandin analogues such as misoprostol, and *H pylori* treatment may also be effective.[53] Women of childbearing age should be warned that misoprostol should be used with caution and may cause fetal demise. Repeat endoscopy and UGI may become necessary to rule out staple line disruption and fistulas for those not healed after 23 months. Intractable disease after 3 months may eventually require a revisional operation.

Any operation involving resection of the stomach is inherently prone to produce postgastrectomy syndromes including dumping, diarrhea, gastric stasis, Roux stasis syndrome, anemia, and bone disease. Most symptoms can successfully be managed medically.

The causes of dumping syndrome are not well known. Early dumping syndrome is believed to be caused by a rapid hyperosmolar load into the small bowel. Absence of a pylorus, highly selective vagotomy, as well as alterations in hormone levels such as vasoactive intestinal peptide and cholecystokinin, contribute to early symptoms. Early dumping may result in diaphoresis, tachycardia, palpitations, and crampy abdominal pain followed by diarrhea. Late dumping is associated with hyperinsulinemia and postprandial reactive hypoglycemia occurring 2 to 3 hours following a meal.[52] Early symptoms may respond to saline infusions. Late symptoms may be relieved by the administration of sugar. Avoidance of liquids during meals, as well as eating small, frequent, high-protein meals, have been described as having good results. For those failing dietary manipulation, medical therapy including octreotide and acarbose may help.[52,54] Most patients improve with medical management. Operative intervention for dumping syndrome has had variable results and long-term follow-up studies are rare.

Diarrhea may occur as an indirect consequence of bariatric surgery. Bacterial overgrowth may occur when the equilibrium between bowel flora and pathogenic bacteria is disturbed. Hydrogen breath tests can confirm bacterial overgrowth, but empiric antibiotic treatment of 7 to 10 days may be cost-effective in aiding diagnosis and treatment.[52] Clinical suspicion should dictate further workup. *Clostridium difficile* infection should be considered as well. Colonoscopy with biopsy should also be considered in refractory diarrhea.

Roux stasis syndrome has been described in patients who have had distal gastrectomy and Roux-en-Y gastrojejunostomy and difficulty with gastric emptying in the absence of obstruction. Patients present with vomiting and epigastric pain. Gastric emptying scans show delayed emptying times. GI motility testing shows abnormal motility in the Roux limb toward the stomach rather than away. The reason why only a subset of patients develop Roux stasis syndrome is unclear. Nevertheless, treatment consists of promotility agents such as metoclopromide, and sometimes serotonergic antidepressants such as mirtazapine, in addition to antiemetics. Severely dilated and flaccid Roux limbs may need resection.[55]

Malabsorption inherently causes a wide variety of nutritional and metabolic effects (**Fig. 7**). Bariatric patients need iron, folate, and B12 (cyanocobalamin) supplementation to prevent iron deficiency and macrocytic anemia. Several case reports have described Wernicke encephalopathy from thiamine (B1) deficiency. Acute psychosis and Wernicke encephalopathy are emergencies that must be treated with thiamine replacement. Multivitamin supplements are also recommended for all bariatric patients. Because of the malabsorptive effect, patients are also at risk for protein deficiency and are instructed to maintain an intake of 60 to 70 g of protein daily.[56] Because of the bypassed segment of bowel containing the biliary limb, fat-soluble vitamins and calcium should be supplemented as well.

Vomiting may have a variety of causes, but good clinical judgment and imaging of the upper GI tract is often required in serious cases to exclude other disorders. IVF resuscitation and electrolyte repletion are important initial maneuvers in treating the vomiting patient. UGI and esophagogastroduodenoscopy are particularly useful to reveal stenosis or ulceration. Suspicion for gastric stasis may warrant gastric emptying studies.[52]

Kidney stone disease has long been associated with malabsorptive bariatric procedures. As fats and calcium are saponified in the gut, an increase in oxalate filtered by the kidney forms calcium oxalate stones. Postsurgical bariatric patients are almost twice as likely as their obese counterparts to develop renal stones. Patients should be warned about this potential complication, which may require lithotripsy or ureteroscopy.[57]

LAPAROSCOPIC SLEEVE GASTRECTOMY

The sleeve gastrectomy is a restrictive operation with resection of the greater curvature of the stomach, theoretically decreasing the amount of the orexigenic hormone ghrelin. Once considered as the preliminary procedure before undergoing biliopancreatic diversion, the sleeve gastrectomy is now feasibly performed by laparoscopy. The efficacy of this operation is comparable with gastric bypass, with similar complication rates, thus reinforcing its usefulness as a stand-alone procedure.[58–61] The ASMBS reviewed a mortality of 0.39% for laparoscopic sleeve gastrectomy and the incidence of complications ranged from 0% to 24%.

Staple line leak rates vary from 0.7% to 3%; it remains the most feared and morbid complication after sleeve gastrectomy and its management remains debatable.[62] Early leaks within 48 hours are believed to be caused by mechanical or technical reasons. Leaks occurring 5 to 7 days later are believed to result from ischemia from tension or poor wound healing. The most common location for leaks is below the gastroesophageal junction, and is believed to be related to the high intragastric

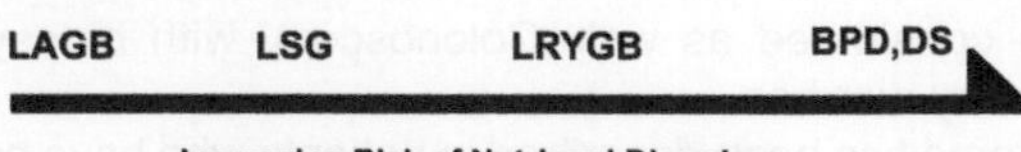

Fig. 7. Relationship of malabsorptive risk among bariatric procedures. (*From* Koch TR, Finelli FC. Postoperative metabolic and nutritional complications of bariatric surgery. Gastroenterol Clin North Am 2010;39:109; with permission.)

pressure coupled with an intact pylorus in addition to impaired distal peristaltic activity and local ischemia. Bovine pericardium has been used to reinforce staple lines with mixed results. Oversewing staple lines has not completely prevented leaks.

When leaks do occur, hemodynamic instability or peritonitis warrant immediate surgical intervention. In stable patients, leaks may be effectively treated with percutaneous drainage and covered esophageal stents.[58–62] Stents are generally removed after 6 weeks. Stents may migrate distally into small bowel, necessitating endoscopic retrieval or, in rare cases, surgery. Endoscopic treatment with fibrin glue and clips has also been described with success for small leaks.

Sleeve strictures are rare but can occur at the incisura and are likely caused by oversewing the staple line. Hematoma and local edema, as well as kinking of the incisura, may contribute to stricture formation. Some surgeons advocate using smaller bougies ranging from 32 to 36F to reduce this incidence. Others advocate using a moderate-sized bougie of 40F with generous oversewing of the staple line.[63]

Weight regain is also a potential complication from incomplete resection because of lack of restriction and retention of gastric cells secreting ghrelin. It is not yet fully known whether gastric dilation in sleeve gastrectomy causes failure to lose weight; however, repeat sleeve gastrectomy or conversion to a combined restrictive/malabsorptive procedure can be considered.[63]

SUMMARY

Like any other surgical specialty, bariatric surgery entails morbidity or mortality. It is important to be knowledgeable in the various complications so that timely and effective measures can be taken to better care for patients. Vague symptoms create diagnostic challenges for this subset of patients, and multidisciplinary care, with a low threshold for exploration, benefits patients. As the bariatric population increases, the educated and decisive first responders will play essential roles in identifying and medically stabilizing ill bariatric patients without delay.

REFERENCES

1. Buchwald H, Avidor Y, Braunwald E, et al. Bariatric surgery: a systematic review and meta-analysis. JAMA 2004;292:1724–37.
2. Fontaine KR, Redden DT, Wang C, et al. Years lost due to obesity. JAMA 2003; 289(2):187–93.
3. Buchwald H, Buchwald JN. Evolution of operative procedures for the management of morbid obesity 1950–2000. Obes Surg 2002;12:705–17.
4. Buchwald H. A bariatric surgery algorithm. Obes Surg 2002;12:733–46.
5. Buchwald H, Estok R, Fahrbach K, et al. Trends in mortality in bariatric surgery: a systematic review and meta-analysis. Surgery 2007;142:621–35.
6. Nguyen NT, Goldman C, Rosenquist CJ, et al. Laparoscopic versus open gastric bypass: a randomized study of outcomes, quality of life, and costs. Ann Surg 2001;234(3):279–91.
7. Parikh MS, Laker S, Weiner M, et al. Objective comparison of complications resulting from laparoscopic bariatric procedures. J Am Coll Surg 2006;202:252–61.
8. Flum DR, Salem L, Elrod JB, et al. Early mortality among Medicare beneficiaries undergoing bariatric surgical procedures. JAMA 2005;294(15):1903–8.
9. Hallowell PT, Stellato TA, Schuster M, et al. Avoidance of complications in older patients and Medicare recipients undergoing gastric bypass. Arch Surg 2007; 142:506–12.

10. Maggard MA, Yermilov T, Li Z, et al. Pregnancy and fertility following bariatric surgery: a systematic review. JAMA 2008;300(19):2286–96.
11. Iavazzo C, Ntziora F, Rousos I, et al. Complications in pregnancy after bariatric surgery. Arch Gynecol Obstet 2010;282:225–7.
12. Levitsky LL, Misra M, Boepple PA, et al. Adolescent obesity and bariatric surgery. Curr Opin Endocrinol Diabetes Obes 2009;16:37–44.
13. Varela JE, Hinojosa MW, Nguyen NT. Perioperative outcomes of bariatric surgery in adolescents compared with adults at academic medical centers. Surg Obes Relat Dis 2007;3:537–42.
14. Spivak H, Favretti F. Avoiding postoperative complications with the LAP-BAND system. Am J Surg 2002;184:31S–7S.
15. Spivak H, Anwar F, Burton S, et al. The LAP-BAND system in the United States. Surg Endosc 2004;18:198–202.
16. Ren CJ, Weiner M, Allen JW. Favorable early results of gastric banding for morbid obesity. Surg Endosc 2004;18:543–6.
17. Carucci LR, Turner MA, Szucs RA. Adjustable laparoscopic gastric banding for morbid obesity: imaging assessment and complications. Radiol Clin North Am 2007;45:261–74.
18. Susmallian S, Ezri T, Elis M, et al. Access-port complications after laparoscopic gastric banding. Obes Surg 2003;13:128–31.
19. Piorkowski JR, Ellner SJ, Mavanur AA, et al. Preventing port site inversion in laparoscopic adjustable gastric banding. Surg Obes Relat Dis 2007;3(2):159–61.
20. Moser F, Gorodner MV, Galvani CA, et al. Pouch enlargement and band slippage: two different entities. Surg Endosc 2006;20:1021–9.
21. Brown WA, Burton PR, Anderson M, et al. Symmetrical pouch dilatation after laparoscopic adjustable gastric banding: incidence and management. Obes Surg 2008;18:1104–8.
22. Keidar A, Szold A, Carmon E, et al. Band slippage after laparoscopic adjustable gastric banding: etiology and treatment. Surg Endosc 2005;19:262–7.
23. Manganiello M, Sarker S, Tempel M, et al. Management of slipped adjustable gastric bands. Surg Obes Relat Dis 2008;4:534–8.
24. Cherian PT, Goussous G, Ashori F, et al. Band erosion after laparoscopic gastric banding: a retrospective analysis of 865 patients over 5 years. Surg Endosc 2010;24(8):2031–8.
25. Higa KD, Boone KB, Ho T. Complications of the laparoscopic Roux-en-Y gastric bypass: 1040 patients-what have we learned? Obes Surg 2000;10:509–13.
26. Carucci LR, Turner MA, Yu J. Imaging evaluation following Roux-en-Y gastric bypass surgery for morbid obesity. Radiol Clin North Am 2007;45:247–60.
27. Mitchell MT. Bariatric imaging: technical aspects and postoperative complications. Appl Radiol 2008;2:10–22.
28. Paroz A, Calmes JM, Giusti V, et al. Internal hernia after laparoscopic Roux-en-Y gastric bypass for morbid obesity: a continuous challenge in bariatric surgery. Obes Surg 2006;16:1482–7.
29. Comeau E, Gagner M, Inabnet WB, et al. Symptomatic internal hernias after laparoscopic bariatric surgery. Surg Endosc 2005;19:34–9.
30. Edwards MA, Jones DB, Ellsmere J, et al. Anastomotic leak following antecolic versus retrocolic laparoscopic roux-en-y gastric bypass for morbid obesity. Obes Surg 2007;17:292–7.
31. Durak E, Inabnet WB, Schrope B, et al. Incidence and management of enteric leaks after gastric bypass for morbid obesity during a 10 year period. Surg Obes Relat Dis 2008;4:389–93.

32. Almahmeed T, Gonzalez R, Nelson LG, et al. Morbidity of anastomotic leaks in patients undergoing Roux-en-Y gastric bypass. Arch Surg 2007;142(10):954–7.
33. Lewis CE, Jensen C, Tejirian T, et al. Early jejunojejunostomy obstruction after laparoscopic gastric bypass: case series and treatment algorithm. Surg Obes Relat Dis 2009;5:203–7.
34. Yu SC, Clapp BL, Lee MJ, et al. Robotic assistance provides excellent outcomes in the learning curve for LRYGB: results from 100 robotic assisted gastric bypasses. Am J Surg 2006;192(6):746–9.
35. Ukleja A, Afonso BB, Pimentel R, et al. Outcomes of endoscopic balloon dilation of strictures after laparoscopic gastric bypass. Surg Endosc 2008; 22:1746–50.
36. Tang S, Olukoga CO, Provost DA, et al. Gastrojejunal stomal reduction with the T-tag device in porcine models (with videos). Gastrointest Endosc 2008;68(1): 132–8.
37. Tang S, Provost DA, Livingston E, et al. Management of transmesenteric tunnel jejunal strictures with endoscopic dilation by using achalasia balloons (with videos). Gastrointest Endosc 2009;70(1):154–8.
38. Prystowsky JB, Morasch MD, Eskandari MK, et al. Prospective analysis of the incidence of deep venous thrombosis in bariatric surgery patients. Surgery 2005;138:759–65.
39. Escalante-Tattersfield T, Tucker O, Fajnwaks P, et al. Incidence of deep vein thrombosis in morbidly obese patients undergoing laparoscopic Roux-en-Y gastric bypass. Surg Obes Relat Dis 2008;4:126–30.
40. Vaziri K, Bhanot P, Hungness ES, et al. Retrievable inferior vena cava filters in high-risk patients undergoing bariatric surgery. Surg Endosc 2009;23:2203–7.
41. Trigilio-Black CM, Ringley CD, McBride CL, et al. Inferior vena cava filter placement for pulmonary embolism risk reduction in super morbidly obese undergoing bariatric surgery. Surg Obes Relat Dis 2007;3:461–4.
42. Melinek J, Livingston E, Cortina G, et al. Autopsy findings following gastric bypass surgery for morbid obesity. Arch Pathol Lab Med 2002;126(9):1091–5.
43. Bakhos C, Alkoury F, Kyriakides T, et al. Early postoperative hemorrhage after open and laparoscopic Roux-en-Y gastric bypass. Obes Surg 2009;19:153–7.
44. Kim JJ, Schirmer B. Safety and efficacy of simultaneous cholecystectomy at Roux-en-Y gastric bypass. Surg Obes Relat Dis 2009;5:48–53.
45. Scott DJ, Villegas L, Sims TL, et al. Intraoperative ultrasound and prophylactic ursodiol for gallstone prevention following laparoscopic gastric bypass. Surg Endosc 2003;17:1796–802.
46. Villegas L, Schneider MD, Provost DA, et al. Is routine cholecystectomy required during laparoscopic gastric bypass? Obes Surg 2004;14:206–11.
47. Hamad GG, Ikramuddin S, Gourash WF, et al. Elective cholecystectomy during laparoscopic Roux-en-Y gastric bypass: is it worth the wait? Obes Surg 2003; 13(1):76–81.
48. Sugerman HJ, Brewer WH, Shiffman ML, et al. A multicenter, placebo-controlled, randomized, double-blind, prospective trial of prophylactic ursodiol for the prevention of gallstone formation following gastric bypass induced rapid weight loss. Am J Surg 1995;169:91–7.
49. Khurana RN, Baudendistel TE, Morgan EF, et al. Postoperative rhabdomyolysis following laparoscopic gastric bypass in the morbidly obese. Arch Surg 2004; 139:73–6.
50. de Oliveira LD, Diniz MT, Diniz M, et al. Rhabdomyolysis after bariatric surgery by Roux-en-Y gastric bypass: a prospective study. Obes Surg 2009;19:1102–7.

51. Stroh C, Hohmann U, Remmler K, et al. Rhabdomyolysis after biliopancreatic diversion with duodenal switch. Obes Surg 2005;15:1347–51.
52. Abell TL, Minocha A. Gastrointestinal complications of bariatric surgery: diagnosis and therapy. Am J Med Sci 2006;331(4):214–8.
53. Sapala JA, Wood MH, Sapala MA, et al. Marginal ulcer after gastric bypass: a prospective 3-year study of 173 patients. Obes Surg 1998;8:505–16.
54. Moreira RO, Moreira RBM, Machado NAM, et al. Post-prandial hypoglycemia after bariatric surgery: pharmacological treatment with verapamil and acarbose. Obes Surg 2008;18:1618–21.
55. Machado JD, Campos CS, Silva CL, et al. Intestinal bacterial overgrowth after Roux-en-Y gastric bypass. Obes Surg 2008;18:139–43.
56. Koch TR, Finelli FC. Postoperative metabolic and nutritional complications of bariatric surgery. Gastroenterol Clin North Am 2010;39:109–24.
57. Matlaga BR, Shore AD, Magnuson T, et al. Effect of gastric bypass surgery on kidney stone disease. J Urol 2009;181:2573–7.
58. Brethauer SA, Hammel JP, Schauer PR. Systematic review of sleeve gastrectomy as staging and primary bariatric procedure. Surg Obes Relat Dis 2009;5:469–75.
59. Frezza EE. Laparoscopic vertical sleeve gastrectomy for morbid obesity. Surg Today 2007;37:275–81.
60. Shi X, Karmali S, Sharma AM, et al. A review of laparoscopic sleeve gastrectomy for morbid obesity. Obes Surg 2010;20(8):1171–7.
61. Cottam D, Qureshi FG, Mattar SG, et al. Laparoscopic sleeve gastrectomy as an initial weight-loss procedure for high-risk patients with morbid obesity. Surg Endosc 2006;20:859–63.
62. Casella G, Soricelli E, Rizzello M, et al. Nonsurgical treatment of staple line leaks after laparoscopic sleeve gastrectomy. Obes Surg 2009;19:821–6.
63. Lalor PF, Tucker ON, Szomstein S, et al. Complications after laparoscopic sleeve gastrectomy. Surg Obes Relat Dis 2008;4:33–8.

Sedation in the Bariatric Patient

John J. Vargo, MD, MPH

KEYWORDS

• Sedation • Obesity • Overweight • Bariatric surgery

Obesity is a significant health problem that has assumed epidemic proportions. The National Health and Nutrition Examination Survey found that over half of the adults in the United States are overweight (body mass index [BMI] >25 kg/m^2).[1] Additionally 32.2% of adults over the age of 20 were found to be obese (BMI >30 kg/m^2), and 4.8% had a BMI greater than 40 kg/m^2.[1] A durable reduction in weight and improved morbidity and mortality have been realized with the introduction of a variety of bariatric surgical procedures. Although controversial, routine preoperative assessment and postoperative bariatric endoscopic assessment are commonly performed. Since certain procedures such as a Roux-en-Y gastric bypass result in the distal stomach or duodenum being inaccessible by a standard upper endoscopy, the threshold for performing a preoperative upper endoscopy is lower. In the postoperative setting, upper endoscopy can help determine the presence of complications such as stenosis or fistula formation.[2] In 2006, approximately 6.25 million colonoscopies were performed in the ambulatory setting.[1] A question that must be answered is whether the current practices of sedation for endoscopic procedures are safe and efficacious in this population. Secondarily, are there any advances in procedural sedation techniques that would prove to be of a particular advantage in patients with morbid obesity? Morbid obesity can result in pulmonary hypertension, obstructive sleep apnea, and restrictive lung disease. In addition, significant alveolar-to-arterial oxygen gradients can develop, which can result in higher supplemental oxygen requirements to maintain adequate arterial oxygenation.[3] This article explores these issues and how they may impact the risk profile of current standards for endoscopic sedation.

ENDOSCOPY SEDATION RISK FACTORS

Does increased BMI equate to an ascendancy of risk during procedural sedation? Intuitively the answer is yes, but this is not backed by extensive data from the literature. Large database-driven studies addressing cardiopulmonary complications during gastrointestinal (GI) endoscopy did not contain BMI in their analyses.[4,5] However other measures such as the American Society of Anesthesiologists (ASA)

Department of Gastroenterology and Hepatology, Digestive Disease Institute, 9500 Euclid Avenue, Desk A-30, Cleveland, OH 44195, USA
E-mail address: vargoj@ccf.org

Gastrointest Endoscopy Clin N Am 21 (2011) 257–263
doi:10.1016/j.giec.2011.02.011
1052-5157/11/$ – see front matter

physical classification score have been found to represent a risk for cardiopulmonary events.[4] In a retrospective study using the Clinical Outcomes Research Initiative database, over 324,737 procedures were reviewed. Multiple logistic regression found that the ASA class was a significant predictor for cardiopulmonary unplanned events. Patients with an ASA class 3 designation exhibited a risk for cardiopulmonary events that was 1.8 times that for the ASA class 1 (odds ratio [OR] 1.8; 95% confidence interval [CI]:1.6–2.0). The risk essentially doubles for each subsequent ASA class thereafter. It should also be emphasized that the calculation of the BMI is simple but has important limitations.[1] For example, extremely muscular patients may fall into the obesity range, whereas patients who have a normal BMI may be nutritionally depleted with a decrease in lean body mass.

Data equating increasing BMI to cardiopulmonary events during endoscopy are available in small case series. A case series of 82 patients undergoing diagnostic upper endoscopy found that a BMI greater than 28 was an independent risk factor for hypoxemia. Qadeer and colleagues[6] found that an increasing BMI was an independent risk factor for hypoxemia in a cohort of 79 subjects undergoing a variety of ambulatory outpatient procedures including upper endoscopy, colonoscopy, endoscopic retrograde cholangiopancreatography (ERCP) and endoscopic ultrasonography (EUS). Other risk factors for hypoxemia included age greater than 60 years and meperidine dose in a study by Dhariwal and colleagues.[7]

The American Society of Anesthesiologists Task Force on Sedation and Analgesia by Nonanesthesiologists stated that there is insufficient published evidence to evaluate the relationship between sedation analgesia outcomes and the performance of a preprocedure patient evaluation. Expert opinion suggested that there is evidence that some pre-existing medical conditions may be related to adverse outcomes in patients receiving either moderate or deep sedation. One of these risk factors is significant obesity, especially involving the neck and facial structures.[8,9] Similarly, the American Gastroenterological Association Institute review of endoscopic sedation recommended the use of an anesthesia professional for patients with morbid obesity.[10] However, this is an expert opinion only, and no evidence was provided for this recommendation. The American Society for Gastrointestinal Endoscopy recommended that a history of sleep apnea, snoring, or stridor should be reviewed as part of the preprocedure assessment.[11]

The presence of obstructive sleep apnea (OSA) has been touted as a risk factor for cardiopulmonary complications for procedural sedation.[8,10,11] Khiani and colleagues[12] used the Berlin Questionnaire, a validated tool for the diagnosis of OSA to determine the incidence of hypoxemia (pulse oximetry <92%) in 233 subjects undergoing elective outpatient upper endoscopy and colonoscopy with targeted moderate sedation using a combination of an opioid and benzodiazepine. Exclusion criteria included a previous diagnosis of OSA, congestive heart failure, chronic obstructive pulmonary disease, long-term narcotic use, haloperidol use or history of substance abuse, and lung disease requiring home oxygen. At the start of the procedure, 2 L of oxygen via nasal cannula was given to all patients. Of the endoscopic procedures performed, 60 (25.8%) patients underwent esophagogastroduodenoscopy (EGD); 155 (66.5%) underwent colonoscopy, and 18 (7.7%) patients underwent both procedures. Thirty-nine percent of the subjects were deemed to be at high risk for OSA by the questionnaire. The high-risk group was significantly older (60.4 plus or minus14.5 vs 55.2 plus or minus 15.2 years, $P<.005$) and exhibited a higher BMI (30.8 plus or minus 5.6 vs 25.9 plus or minus 4.7 kg/m^2, $P<.001$). There was no difference between the groups in terms of age, gender, ethnicity, or mean medication dosage. There was no significant difference in the rate of transient hypoxia between the high- and low-risk groups (OR 1.48; 95% CI 0.58–3.80). Important caveats can be gleaned from this study:

There was no stratification between upper endoscopy and colonoscopy. It is felt that orally intubated subjects are at higher risk for cardiopulmonary events.

This was a relatively healthy cohort of patients, and in the setting of relatively brief procedures targeting moderate sedation, there appears to be a minimal risk in subjects felt to be at risk for OSA.

Does snoring during moderate sedation predict OSA? Sharara and colleagues[13] studied 131 subjects undergoing elective ambulatory colonoscopy. Each completed a detailed sleep questionnaire and physical examination focused on detecting OSA (BMI, neck circumference, and the presence of craniofacial abnormalities). Subjects who snored during colonoscopy in the left lateral decubitus position for at least 10 seconds were referred for nocturnal polysomnography. Gender- and BMI-matched patients who did not snore served as controls. All subjects who snored during colonoscopy exhibited a significantly higher Mallampati score and greater BMI and neck circumference and were more likely to report daytime sleepiness than controls. Portable nocturnal polysomnography diagnosed OSA in all snoring subjects compared with only 4 of 18 controls (P<.001).

SEDATION OPTIONS

Numerous case series have been published involving elective upper endoscopy and the preoperative and postoperative assessments of bariatric surgery patients.[14–17] Frequently, the medications administered were the combination of the opioid and a benzodiazepine. Unfortunately, cardiopulmonary endpoints and patient tolerance were not that the focus of these articles. For example, Catalano and colleagues[18] performed endoscopic balloon dilation of anastomotic stenosis in 26 consecutive patients with a prior Roux-en-Y gastric bypass for morbid obesity. The patients received moderate sedation with the combination of meperidine and midazolam. Although no specific cardiopulmonary endpoints were described, no procedure related complications were seen during the course of the dilating. To the author's knowledge, there is no prospective trial comparing the safety of monitored anesthesia care (MAC) with endoscopist-directed sedation in subjects undergoing GI endoscopy. The ASA closed claims project compared MAC with general anesthesia for injury- and liability-associated claims.[19] Respiratory depression after an absolute or relative overdose of medication was the most common cause for adverse events in the MAC group. Nearly half of the MAC claims were judged to be preventable with better monitoring and improve vigilance.

One-hundred subjects undergoing routine preoperative assessment before bariatric surgery received either monitored anesthesia care with propofol versus a combination of narcotic and benzodiazepine administered by a surgical endoscopist.[20] There were no significant differences between the two sedation arms with respect to subjective assessment of recovery in postprocedure recall. This study was hampered by the fact that it was not randomized, and a phone survey was used 1 to 3 months following the procedure.

Is monitored anesthesia care without risk? Coté and colleagues[21] studied 231 consecutive patients undergoing advanced procedures such as ERCP and endoscopic ultrasound with anesthesiologist-directed propofol sedation. A previously validated screening tool for OSA known as the snore, tired, obstruction, pressure -BMI, age, neck, gender (STOP -BANG) (SB) questionnaire was used to identify patients at high risk for OSA. This screening tool uses questions such as the occurrence of snoring as well as physiologic measurements such as a BMI. A score greater than or equal to 3 out of 8 is indicative of an increased risk for OSA. The incidence airway maneuvers such as a chin lift, placement of nasopharyngeal airway, bag mask ventilation, and endotracheal intubation were tallied between the SB-positive and SB-negative subjects. Other significant adverse events such as hypoxemia, hypotension apnea, and early procedure termination due to a cardiovascular event were tallied. SB-positive subjects were more likely to exhibit hypoxemia and require an airway intervention when compared with SB-negative subjects. This difference remained significant after adjusting for an ASA physiologic class 3 or higher. This study shows that a risk stratification for OSA can be helpful in identifying patients who may require airway maneuvers during anesthesiologist-directed propofol sedation for advanced endoscopic procedures. Further data are needed regarding gastroenterologist-directed sedation for procedures not requiring deep sedation, as well as those requiring general anesthesia.

Are there any alternative forms of procedural sedation that may benefit the obese patient? Dexmedetomidine is a highly selective α_2 adrenal receptor antagonist that possesses hypnotic, sedative, anxiolytic, and analgesic properties. A unique aspect of this medication is that it does not produce significant respiratory depression and hence may be of advantage in obese subjects undergoing endoscopic procedures.[22,23] Disadvantages of this medication include the fact that a loading dose coupled with an infusion is necessary. Moreover, it is not released for use by non-anesthesiologists. The use of this agent during operative procedures has been shown to be of benefit. A case report described the utility of this medication in a morbidly obese patient undergoing a Roux-en- y gastric bypass.[24] Eighty ASA 2 to 3 patients underwent laparoscopic bariatric surgery with the use of dexmedetomidine.[25] In this randomized double-blind placebo-controlled dose ranging study, dexmedetomidine was found to lead to a significantly faster emergence from anesthesia with no significant difference in the intraoperative hemodynamic parameters.

In a prospective randomized trial, patients undergoing elective outpatient colonoscopy were randomized to 4 sedation regimens including dexmedetomidine, meperidine with midazolam, and fentanyl on demand.[26] Primary outcomes included cardiorespiratory parameters, as well as recovery time. The study was terminated early due to the side effects stemming from dexmedetomidine. A randomized trial compared the safety and efficacy of dexmedetomidine versus midazolam for 50 ASA 2 to 3 adults undergoing elective upper endoscopy.[27] There were no difference between the 2 sedation arms with respect to heart rate and mean arterial pressure. Patient satisfaction was significantly higher in the dexmedetomidine group. A small randomized trial compared the combination of propofol to dexmedetomidine for elective ERCP.[28] Dexmedetomidine was not was found not to be as effective as the combination of fentanyl and propofol for conscious sedation. As in previous endoscopic studies, it was also found to be limited due to hemodynamic instability.

Another alternative to sedated procedures would be transnasal small-caliber endoscopes. Alami and colleagues[29] used this method in 25 morbidly obese subjects undergoing a preoperative upper endoscopy. The average BMI was 47 (range 38–69 kg/m^2). Sixty-eight percent of the patients had a history of OSA. No sedation was required for 23 of the patients. Pathology was identified in 14 of the 25 patients including Barrett esophagus, gastric polyps, esophageal varices, and gastric ulcers. Biopsies were successful in 12 out of 12 patients. No data were presented regarding hemodynamic parameters or patient tolerance.

EMERGING SEDATION TECHNOLOGIES

Patient-controlled sedation and analgesia (PCSA) allows for a customized approach to procedural sedation. Typically, a specialized pump delivers a predetermined bolus dose of medication. A lockout interval is used to prevent oversedation. An infusion may or may not be used. Important prerequisites are that the targeted level of sedation is moderate sedation and it requires a cooperative patient. Patients requiring deep sedation or general anesthesia are not candidates for this type of sedation delivery. PCSA usually involves the administration of a rapidly acting narcotic coupled with propofol. Most data reside in patients undergoing colonoscopy. There are no studies in obese subjects. Recovery time is usually improved when compared with standard sedation with equivalent to improved satisfaction and no appreciable difference in cardiopulmonary parameters.[30,31]

Target controlled infusion (TCI) typically involves a computer-aided infusion of sedation agents that is designed to result in a steady-state effect site drug concentration. This is based on pharmacologic modeling. Since this is population-based, variances in the response can be expected, and adjustments in the infusion rate are accomplished by some type of physiologic feedback such as by bipsectral index monitoring (closed loop) or via the physician (open loop). As opposed to patient-controlled sedation, TCI can be cut targeted to deeper levels of sedation for extended intervals. A case series by Gillham and colleagues[32] exhibited a 15% rate of undersedation and a 20% rate of oversedation using TCI. A much larger study by Fanti and colleagues[33] used target controlled propofol infusion during monitored anesthesia in patients undergoing ERCP. Excellent sedation was seen in 201 of the 205 patients. Stonell and colleagues[34] compared anesthesiologist-administered propofol sedation with patient-controlled sedation using effect site steering with propofol. Endoscopist and patient satisfaction were similar between the two sedation arms.

Computer-assisted personalized sedation (CAPS) is a form of target controlled infusion that theoretically enables the nonanesthesiologist administration of propofol targeting moderate sedation. The platform uses both an infusion and bolus administration of propofol. Physiologic feedback includes capnography, pulse oximetry, electrocardiography, and blood pressure monitoring. In addition, automated responsiveness monitoring is employed, which measures the patient's ability to respond to tactile or and auditory stimulation. A multicenter study involving 1000 patients undergoing elective upper endoscopy and colonoscopy has recently been published.[35] Subjects were randomized to receive either standard sedation with the combination of an opioid and benzodiazepine or sedation with the CAPS device. Patients with a BMI between 30 kg/m^2 and 35 kg/m^2 were enrolled but not targeted for a specific analysis. Subjects in the CAPS arm exhibited significantly less hypoxemia and improved recovery times when compared with standard sedation.

SUMMARY

In summary, the approach to procedural endoscopic sedation in the obese patient remains one of expert opinion with very little data to guide the clinician. Clearly an increasing BMI carries with it some measure of cardiopulmonary risk. There is currently no way to quantify this risk. Numerous case series point to the effectiveness of the combination of an opioid and benzodiazepine for elective upper endoscopic procedures. It is important to point out that the target for these procedures is almost always moderate sedation. For those cases in which deeper levels of sedation are needed or a longer endoscopic procedure is planned, such as ERCP or EUS, the use of anesthesiologist support seems prudent. There is no substitute for a clinician who is well aware of the physiology of the patient, and the pharmacokinetics and adverse effects of the agents available for sedation. Future advances in this challenging group of patients are eagerly awaited.

REFERENCES

1. Defining overweight and obesity. Available at: http://www.cdc.gov/obesity/defining.html. Accessed January 30, 2011.
2. ASGE Standards of Practice Committee. Role of endoscopy in the bariatric patient. Gastrointest Endosc 2008;68:1–10.
3. Sugarman HJ. Pulmonary function in morbid obesity. Gastroenterol Clin North Am 1987;16:225–37.
4. Sharma VK, Nguyen CC, Crowell MD, et al. A national study of cardiopulmonary unplanned events after GI endoscopy. Gastrointest Endosc 2007;66:27–34.
5. Gangi S, Saidi F, Patel K, et al. Cardiovascular complications after GI endoscopy: occurrence and risks in a large hospital system. Gastrointest Endosc 2004;60: 679–85.
6. Qadeer MA, Lopez R, Dumot JA, et al. Risk factors for hypoxemia during in dilatory gastrointestinal endoscopy in ASA I-II patients. Dig Dis Sci 2009;54:1035–40.
7. Dhariwal A, Plevris JV, Lo NT, et al. Age anemia and obesity associated oxygen desaturation during upper gastrointestinal endoscopy. Gastrointest Endosc 1992;38:684–8.
8. Gross JB, Bailey PL, Connis RT, et al. Practice guidelines for sedation and analgesia by nonanesthesiologists. Anesthesiology 2002;96:1004–17.
9. Metzner J, Posner KL, Domino KB. The risk and safety of anesthesia at remote locations: the US closed claims analysis. Curr Opin Anaesthesiol 2009;22:502–8.
10. Cohen LB, DeLegge MH, Aisenberg J, et al. AGA Institute review of endoscopic sedation. Gastroenterology 2007;133:675–701.
11. ASGE Standards of Practice Committee. Sedation and anesthesia in GI endoscopy. Gastrointest Endosc 2008;68:205–16.
12. Khiani VJ, Salah W, Cummings L, et al. Sedation for patients at risk of obstructive sleep apnea. Gastrointest Endosc 2009;70:1116–20.
13. Sharara AI, El Zahabi L, Maasri K, et al. Persistent snoring under conscious sedation during colonoscopy is a predictor of obstructive sleep apnea. Gastrointest Endosc 2010;71:1224–30.
14. Madan AK, Speck KE, Hiller NL. Routine preoperative upper endoscopy for laparoscopic gastric bypass: is it necessary? Am Surg 2004;70:684–6.
15. Verset D, Houben JJ, Gay F, et al. The place of upper gastrointestinal tract endoscopy before and after vertical banded gastroplasty for morbid obesity. Dig Dis Sci 1997;42:2333–7.
16. Shirmer B, Erenoglu C, Miller A. Flexible endoscopy in the management of patients undergoing roux-en- Y gastric bypass. Obes Surg 2002;12:634–8.
17. Barbara CA, Butensky CA, Lorenzo M, et al. Endoscopic dilation of gastroesophageal anastomotic stricture after gastric bypass. Surg Endosc 2003;17:416–20.
18. Catalano MF, Chua TY, Rudic G. Endoscopic balloon dilation of stomal stenosis following gastric bypass. Obes Surg 2007;17:298–303.
19. Bhanaker SM, Posner KL, Cheney FW, et al. Injury and liability associated with monitored anesthesia care. Anesthesiology 2006;104:228–34.
20. Madan AK, Tichnasky DS, Isom J, et al. Monitored anesthesia care with propofol versus surgeon- monitored sedation with benzodiazepines in narcotics for preoperative endoscopy in the morbidly obese. Obes Surg 2008;18:545–8.

21. Coté GA, Hovis CE, Hovis RM, et al. A screening instrument for sleep apnea predicts airway maneuvers in patients undergoing advanced endoscopic procedures. Clin Gastroenterol Hepatol 2010;108:660–5.
22. Antaa R, Scheinin M. A2 Alpha-2 adrenergic agents in anesthesia. Acta Anaesthesiol Scand 1993;37:1–16.
23. Bloor BC, Ward DS, Belleville JP, et al. Effects of IV dexmedetomidine in humans: II hemodynamic changes. Anesthesiology 1992;77:1134–42.
24. Hofer RE, Sprung J, Sarr MG, et al. Anesthesia for a patient with morbid obesity using dexmedetomidine without narcotics. Can J Anaesth 2005;52:176–80.
25. Tufanogullari B, White PF, Peixoto MP, et al. Dexmedetomidine infusion during laparoscopic bariatric surgery: the effect on recovery outcome variables. Anesth Analg 2008;106:1741–8.
26. Jalowiecki P, Rudner R, Gonciarz M, et al. Sole use of dexmedetomidine has limited use for conscious sedation during outpatient colonoscopy. Anesthesiology 2005;103:269–73.
27. Demiraran Y, Korkut E, Tamer A, et al. The comparison of dexmedetomidine and midazolam used for sedation of patients during upper endoscopy: a prospective randomized study. Can J Gastroenterol 2007;21:25–9.
28. Mueller S, Borowics SM, Fortis EA, et al. Clinical efficacy of dexmedetomidine alone is less than propofol for conscious sedation during ERCP. Gastrointest Endosc 2008;67:651–9.
29. Alami RS, Schuster R, Friedland S, et al. Transnasal small-caliber esophagogastroduodenoscopy for preoperative evaluation of high-risk morbidly obese patients. Surg Endosc 2007;21:758–60.
30. Bright E, Roseveare C, Dalgleisch D, et al. Patient controlled sedation for colonoscopy: a randomized trial comparing patient-controlled administration of propofol and alfentanil with physician-administered midazolam and pethidine. Endoscopy 2003;35:63–7.
31. Heuss LT, Drewe J, Schnieper P, et al. Patient controlled versus nurse administered sedation for colonoscopy: a prospective randomized trial. Am J Gastroenterol 2004;9:515–8.
32. Gillham MJ, Hutchinson RC, Carter R, et al. Patient maintained sedation for ERCP with a target controlled infusion of propofol: a pilot study. Gastrointest Endosc 2001;54:14–7.
33. Fanti L, Agostoni M, Casta A, et al. Target controlled propofol infusion during monitored anesthesia in patients undergoing ERCP. Gastrointest Endosc 2004; 60:361–6.
34. Stonell A, Leslie K, Absalom AR. Effect site target targeted patient controlled sedation with propofol: comparison with anesthesiologist administration for colonoscopy. Anaesthesia 2006;61:240–7.
35. Pambianco DJ, Vargo JJ, Pruitt RE, et al. Computer-assisted personalized sedation for upper endoscopy and colonoscopy: a comparative, multicenter randomized study. Gastrointest Endosc 2010. [Epub ahead of print].

Endoscopy Unit Considerations in the Care of Obese Patients

Gregory G. Ginsberg, MD*, Octavia Pickett-Blakely, MD, MHS

KEYWORDS

• Bariatric • Endoscopy • Endoscopy unit
• Gastrointestinal endoscopy • Bariatric endoscopy

The prevalence of class III obesity (body mass index >40 kg/m^2) has increased dramatically. As such, bariatric surgery procedures have increased, with surgery becoming widely accepted as the most effective method of weight loss for severe obesity. Gastrointestinal endoscopy has a role in preoperative patient assessment, management of postoperative complications, and as a potential initial bariatric treatment with emerging endoscopic bariatric therapies. Endoscopy units should address the unique design and equipment needs of obese patients in both their short-range and long-range planning. Obese patients require more health care resources than nonobese patients, and there are greater physical challenges for staff and attendants administering care to obese individuals. Basic patient transfer is one such example. Bariatric patients encompass a wide weight range, from roughly 250 to 300 lbs (113–136 kg) to more than 1200 lbs (544 kg). Transferring bariatric patients of these different weight ranges may require special techniques, equipment, and training to assure safety of both the patients and the health care professionals.

Safe and effective performance of gastrointestinal endoscopy has the following requirements (**Table 1**):

- An adequately trained and credentialed endoscopist to perform specific gastrointestinal endoscopic procedures
- Properly trained nursing and ancillary personnel
- Operational, well-maintained equipment
- Adequately designed and equipped space for patient preparation, performance of procedures, and patient recovery

Gastroenterology Division, Hospital of the University of Pennsylvania, 3rd Floor Ravdin Building, 3400 Spruce Street, Philadelphia, PA 19104, USA
* Corresponding author.
E-mail address: gregory.ginsberg@uphs.upenn.edu

Gastrointest Endoscopy Clin N Am 21 (2011) 265–274
doi:10.1016/j.giec.2011.02.013 giendo.theclinics.com
1052-5157/11/$ – see front matter

Table 1
Endoscopy unit considerations

All Endoscopy Facilities	Facilities Catering to Obese Patients
A properly trained endoscopist with appropriate privileges to perform specific gastrointestinal endoscopic procedures	The facility should comply with the standards of the Americans with Disabilities Act
Properly trained nursing and ancillary personnel	Staff must be experienced with and sensitive to the special needs of bariatric patients, and protected against ergonomic and lifting injuries Staffing must be sufficient to safely care for the bariatric patient
Operational, well-maintained equipment	Specially rated procedure tables (stretchers) for patients with morbid and supermorbid obesity Carbon dioxide insufflation should be available for endoscopic retrograde cholangiopancreatography and deep enteroscopy procedures
Adequately designed and equipped space for patient preparation, performance of procedures, and patient recovery	Facility sized for passage of large-capacity rolling stretchers and wheelchairs through doorways and passages Generously appointed common areas (waiting room, bathroom, etc), with appropriately sized furniture and reinforced commodes, should be available for bariatric patients and their family members
Trained personnel and appropriate equipment to perform cardiopulmonary resuscitation	Access to anesthesia providers is desirable Ambulances servicing free-standing endoscopy centers must be equipped to safely care for bariatric patients

- Trained personnel and appropriate equipment to perform cardiopulmonary resuscitation.

Moreover, for bariatric patients, the following additional considerations apply:

- Facility compliance with the standards of the Americans with Disabilities Act[1]
- A generously appointed waiting room to accommodate bariatric patients and their family members
- Appropriately sized endoscopy unit for passage of large-capacity rolling stretchers and wheelchairs through doorways and passages
- Specially rated procedure tables (stretchers) for patients with severe obesity
- Staff experienced with and sensitive to the special needs of bariatric patients, and protected against ergonomic and lifting injuries.[2]

This article details endoscopy unit considerations pertaining to the bariatric patient, which may apply to pretreatment endoscopic evaluation, postoperative management of bariatric surgical complications, and emerging endoluminal bariatric therapies.

TYPE OF FACILITY

Endoscopy facilities vary, and include hospital-based endoscopy units, single-specialty or multispecialty ambulatory surgery centers (ASCs), and office-based endoscopy suites. Each model has its unique set of advantages, disadvantages, and regulatory issues. The hospital and ASC environments are highly regulated by state and federal agencies and third-party accreditation bodies. In the United States these include the Joint Commission on Accreditation of Healthcare Organizations (JCAHO), the Accreditation Association for Ambulatory Healthcare (AAAHC), and the American Association for Accreditation of Ambulatory Surgery Facilities (AAAASF). Private payers sometimes impose their own specific requirements. Office endoscopy suites, previously less regulated, have been subject to more control by state and federal agencies in recent years.

The institutional needs of a bariatric program extend across outpatient and inpatient environments. The American Society for Metabolic and Bariatric Surgery (ASMBS) has established a Bariatric Surgery Centers of Excellence program. Education and guidance documents are managed by the independent Surgical Review Corporation (SRC). The Bariatric Surgery Review Committee (BSRC) reviews the information, determines whether the guidelines are met, and grants or denies the designation. Many of these principles may be applied to endoscopy units serving the needs of bariatric patients, and in particular for units being developed to perform emerging endoluminal bariatric procedures. Provisional Status requires evidence of an institutional commitment to excellence in the care of bariatric patients, as demonstrated by infrastructure investment and ongoing in-service education programs in the management of bariatric patients.

Hospitals with established bariatric surgery programs are expected to have these provisions in place, at least within dedicated auspices. When performing endoscopic procedures on hospitalized bariatric patients it is desirable to make use of existing provisions; this may mean performing endoscopic procedures in existing bariatric operating room space, and may be the best course of action for managing the superobese and acutely ill patients in the perioperative period. In the former group, facilities and staff dedicated to their management may prove necessary. In most other circumstances, existing endoscopic facilities should be modified and new facilities developed to accommodate bariatric patients, at least within a component of their functionality.

GENERAL CONSIDERATIONS

Endoscopy units caring for bariatric patients should be expected to maintain a full line of equipment and instruments for the care of such patients.[2] Radiologic tables and facilities for fluoroscopic imaging of obese patients are also desirable. These requirements apply to management of postoperative strictures, leaks and fistulas, and postoperative pancreaticobiliary endoscopy. In addition, these technologies are apt to play roles in emerging endoluminal bariatric procedures.

Most programs currently do not have separate endoscopy units for bariatric patients. In the past, the occasional severely obese patient was handled on an ad hoc basis with existing equipment. Endoscopy programs should have access to equipment and instruments for the care of patients who undergo bariatric surgery. Such equipment may include bariatric procedure tables, lifts, accessories (eg, clips, stents, fibrin glue), and fluoroscopy apparatus to accommodate class III obesity. Radiology equipment with a weight capacity of more than 450 lbs (200 kg) has only recently become available. In addition, chairs, beds, scales, floor-mounted or supported toilets, wheelchairs, and stretchers/litters that are strong enough and wide enough to accommodate the severely obese are required. Furniture and equipment should be able to accommodate patients who are within the anticipated patient weight limits established by the program. Weight capacities should be documented by the manufacturer's specifications, and this information should be available to relevant staff.[3]

In accordance with provisional status designation by the SRC, appropriate patient movement/transfer systems must also be located wherever bariatric surgery patients receive care. Personnel must be trained to use the equipment and, most importantly, be capable of moving these individuals without injury to the patient or themselves. That said, hospital-based and ambulatory endoscopy units do not need to change all of the equipment, furniture, and instruments throughout the entire facility. This requirement only applies to those areas where patients undergoing bariatric surgery receive care. For some programs, then, this is a dedicated bariatric patient care area. Endoscopic outcomes may well be enhanced when conducted by endoscopists and in endoscopy units with a particular interest, investment, and higher volume of bariatric and related endoscopy.

Reception Area

Severe obesity is associated with social stigma and discrimination. Therefore, obese individuals are often reluctant to venture out of their homes and comfort zones. There are many factors for consideration in the shaping of a space to accommodate severely obese patients—some patently evident, and others that are less obvious. It is important to have furniture, clothing, doorways, bathrooms, and wheelchairs that are appropriate and comfortable for patients with severe obesity and for their families. Families of obese patients tend to be large-sized also, and accommodations for accompanying family members must also be considered (**Fig. 1**).

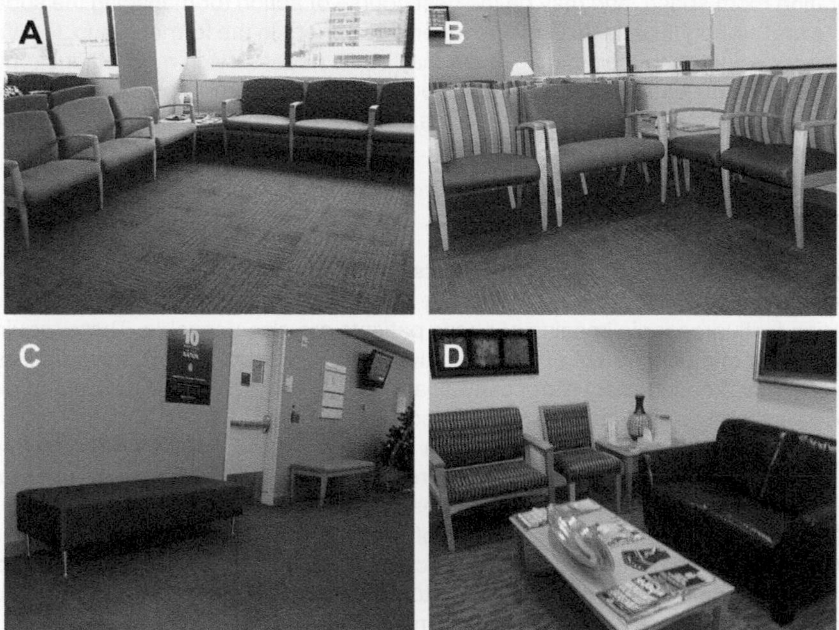

Fig. 1. (*A–D*) Reception area seating should make use of reinforced and large-capacity chairs, couches, and bench seating that will be safe, dignified, and comfortable for morbidly obese patients. Families of obese patients tend to be large-sized also, so accommodations for accompanying family members must also be considered.

Preparation/Recovery Area

Larger beds and larger equipment necessitate larger room dimensions, but planners must recognize that the main determinant of more space is the need for clearance around furniture and equipment to allow the care team to maneuver.

Because severely obese patients, many weighing upwards of 500 lbs (227 kg) and some approaching 1000 lbs (454 kg) are more than one nurse can handle, there must always be at least 2 in the care team to assist in patient transfers and positioning. There are instances when 3 or more caregivers are recommended for patient handling. In addition, extra-large blood pressure cuffs are an essential accessory for monitoring extremely obese patients.

Patient and staff safety should be factored into endoscopy unit design. Employing proper ergonomic techniques is critical to ensuring safety for the care team when assisting the patient. Ergonomically sound transfer techniques require ample clearance at the bedside and in patient seating zones. Furthermore, transferring these patients often requires the use of lifts, yet another reason for ample clearance around the bed.

Even with the most observant and cautious care, patients may fall. Undesired consequences when the severely obese patient falls are notably increased. Wide spacing between the bed and other obstacles will facilitate the care team's effort in up righting the patient. Wide spacing of furniture and equipment can mitigate the probability of the patient striking objects during a fall.

According to Pelczarski,[4] among the most significant facility design flaws are inadequate doorway widths. Doorways that are too narrow (eg, 34 in [864 mm]) may be problematic for ambulatory bariatric patients using an assistive device such as a walker. Narrow doorways may also be problematic for nonambulatory bariatric patients. Bariatric wheelchairs can be up to 39 inches (991 mm) wide while bariatric beds and stretchers may expand to 57 inches (1448 cm) wide with the side rails up.

The *Guidelines for Design and Construction of Hospital and Health Care Facilities* set forth by the American Institute of Architects (AIA) mandate a minimum of 3 ft (915 mm) for clearances around the patient bed in a single room. Through a trial of pushing bariatric wheelchairs, stretchers, and beds around in a mock-up room, one group of experts recommended a 5-ft (1524 mm) clearance on the sides and at the foot of the bed.[5] This ensures adequate clearance for the care team to assist the patient in and out of the room or to the bathroom. To accommodate a patient with a bariatric walker and allow passage for other foot traffic, a minimum of 5 ft (60 in or 1524 mm) is required for the width of a corridor (**Fig. 2**).[6]

To accommodate bariatric wheelchairs, 45-inch (1143 mm) doorway openings are required. Where the passage of bariatric stretchers is needed, doorways should be a minimum of 52 inches (1320 mm).[5] The door to the procedure room needs to be congruent with the larger room clearances. A width of 60 inches is considered sufficient to allow comfortable passage of oversized equipment.

Bathroom Facilities

The AIA recommends floor-mounted toilets with a drop weight rating of 700 lbs (317.5 kg) (to accommodate an impact factor of 1.4 for a 500-lb [227 kg] patient) and a clearance of 5 ft (60 in or 1520 mm).[5] These dimensions allow for staff assistance on both sides of the toilet if needed. Wall-mounted sinks with a rating of 300 lbs (136 kg) are recommended because floor-mounted sinks interfere with wheelchairs. Lastly, the AIA recommends that all walls containing a wall-mounted fixture be reinforced to meet or exceed the rating.

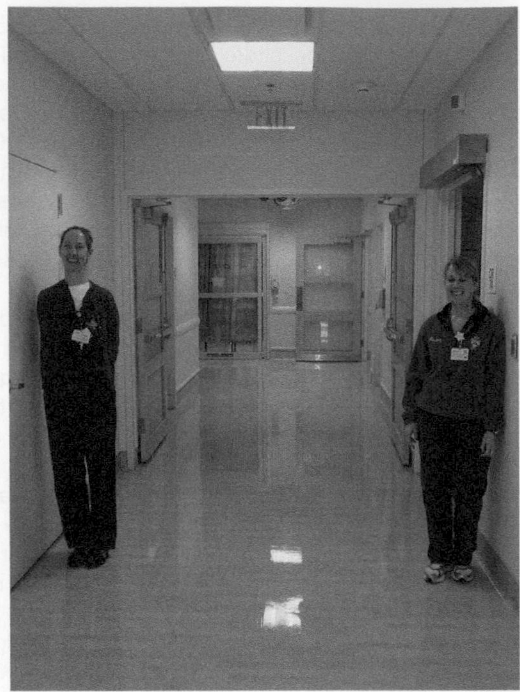

Fig. 2. To accommodate a patient with a bariatric walker and allow passage for other foot traffic, a minimum of 5 ft (60 in or 1520 mm) is required for the width of a corridor.

Procedure Room Size

The minimum size for a typical endoscopy room is approximately 300 square feet, to accommodate videoendoscopy equipment, video monitors, and additional equipment for anesthesia services.[7,8] Some state licensing departments or Medicare services will mandate a minimum size for an "operating room" that may best accommodate the bariatric patient. The AIA *Guidelines for Design and Construction of Hospital and Health Care Facilities*, 2001 Edition, states that for "surgical suites for special procedures that require additional personnel and/or large equipment, the room shall have … a minimum clear area of 600 square feet, with a minimum of 20 feet clear dimension …."[6] Such is the expectation for a bariatric operating room in which open operative procedures are performed, and which would clearly be excessive for endoscopic bariatric procedures.

An example of an endoscopy procedure room layout is shown in **Fig. 3**, which shows placement of the light source, video processor, electrosurgical generator, vacuum, and gases on a ceiling-mounted boom. Dual video monitors articulate from ceiling-mounted booms. This arrangement provides flexibility in room orientation to facilitate many procedure and patient types. The patient enters and exits on a procedural stretcher cart. The floor is largely free of cables and wiring, these being arranged above via dropped ceiling and the ceiling-mounted booms. This system allows patients, physicians, staff, and equipment to move about unfettered by cords and cables, and avoids damaging these sensitive components. Doors are automated from wall-mounted sensors.

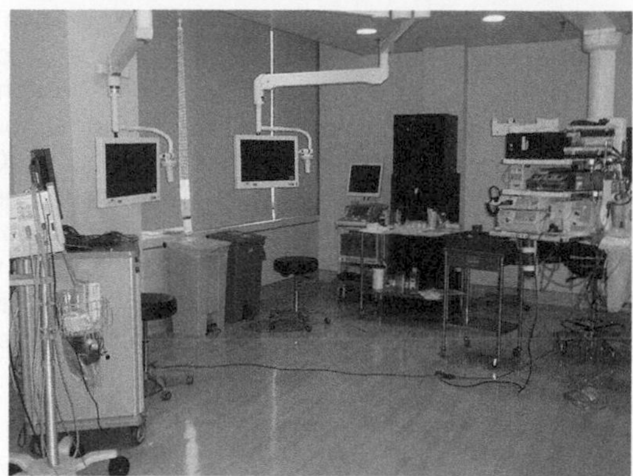

Fig. 3. The endoscopy procedure room should be a minimum of 300 square feet. Ideally the light source, video processor, and so forth are placed on a ceiling-mounted boom. Dual video monitors also articulate from ceiling-mounted booms. This arrangement provides flexibility in room orientation to facilitate a variety of procedure and patient types.

Procedure Tables

In general, procedure tables are being replaced by height-adjustable rolling procedural stretcher carts that allow patients, once properly gowned for endoscopy, to mount the moveable cart and not leave it until ready to leave the facility. These useful carts allow patients to be shuttled from preparation areas to procedure rooms and back to recovery areas, and serve as procedure tables. This capability is very important to overall system efficiency, and adds to patient safety by avoiding transfer to and from a procedure table. A battery-powered stretcher chair that converts from an upright mobile chair to a prone, stretcher position with an infinite number of positions in between is very useful (**Fig. 4**). Available bariatric transfer chairs allow a single caregiver to safely and easily transfer limited or nonambulatory patients, with seat widths up to 27 inches (686 mm) and weight capacity up to 700 lbs (317.5 kg).

Endoscopic Equipment

Endoscopic bariatric procedures for the treatment of obesity are emerging. At present, intragastric balloons are being used in some countries as a restrictive method for

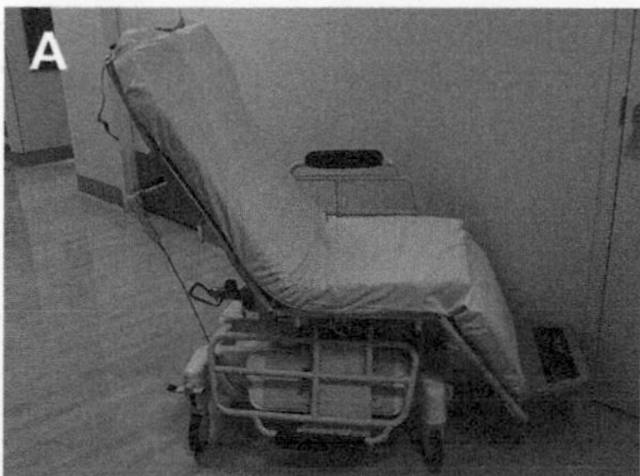

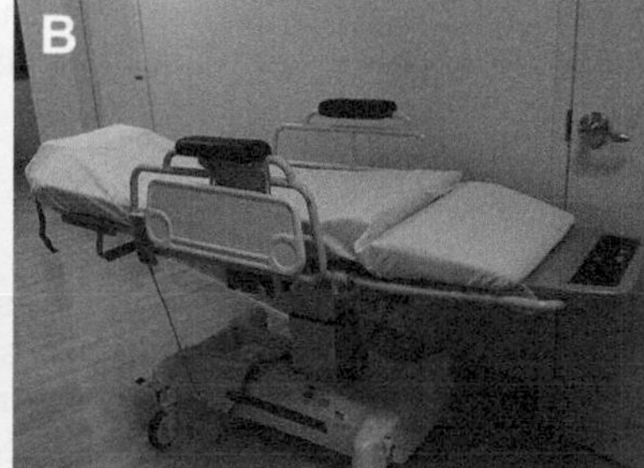

Fig. 4. (*A, B*) This battery-powered stretcher chair converts from an upright mobile chair to a prone stretcher position with an infinite number of positions in between. Available bariatric models allow a single caregiver to safely and easily transfer limited or nonambulatory patients, with seat widths up to 27 inches (686 mm) and weight capacity up to 700 lbs (317.5 kg).

short-term weight loss. Endoscopic suturing and plication devices are being developed and investigated as restrictive options for weight loss. Endoluminal bypass sleeves may yield successful weight loss by inducing malabsorption and/or improvement in metabolic parameters in obese patients. Although endoscopic bariatric procedures are promising, currently the Roux-en-Y gastric bypass (RYGBP) is the most commonly performed surgical bariatric procedure. Diagnostic endoscopy is often indicated during the preoperative evaluation before bariatric surgery. Postoperative complications and revisions are increasingly being managed with endoscopic therapies.[9] Although endoscopic management of biliopancreatic disorders is readily accessible in patients with unaltered anatomy, the postoperative anatomy poses unique challenges to endoscopic evaluation and management.

Scopes

For most patients with RYGBP, a standard gastroscope is sufficient to evaluate the esophagus, gastric pouch, gastrojejunal anastomosis, and proximal portion of the alimentary limb. A pediatric-caliber colonoscope or dedicated enteroscope may be required to evaluate the jejunojejunal anastomosis. More recently, balloon-assisted enteroscopy (dedicated double-balloon and single-balloon systems) and related adjuncts (spiral overtube and balloon catheter mediated) facilitate examination of the biliopancreatic limb, the excluded stomach, and diagnostic and therapeutic endoscopic retrograde cholangiopancreatography (ERCP). Preoperative investigation may be undertaken with unsedated endoscopy using an ultrathin transnasal endoscope. This procedure can be performed with the patient seated in a wheelchair and topical anesthetic, thus avoiding the need for intravenous sedation.

Accessories

Apart from ordinary endoscopic accessories, endoscopy for management of post-RYGBP and other bariatric surgeries may employ a variety of endoscopic clips, dilators, stents, sealants, and thermal and abrasive devices. Management of postoperative leaks may be particularly rewarding. Chronic fistulae are more challenging and may benefit from incorporation of biomaterial tissue plugs. Operators should be cognizant of off-label use of stents and biomaterials in these settings, and ensure full disclosure as a component of risk management.

The ampullary orifice can be accessed in patients following RYGBP with device-assisted enteroscopy. Currently available therapeutic enteroscopes will accept accessories of standard colonoscope length. Devices for cannulation, sphincterotomy, stone extraction, and stent therapies should be made available in preparation for such procedures. Carbon dioxide gas insufflation appears to reduce postprocedural gas, bloating, and discomfort following ERCP and deep enteroscopy procedures. Therefore, it should be made available for device-assisted enteroscopy-mediated ERCP in post-RYGBP patients.

STAFF

Sensitivity training and education for endoscopy staff should be provided in an effort to foster a culture of respect and compassion for obese patients. Endoscopy staff must be able to appreciate the morbidity associated with class III obesity.[3] Staffing models should be developed and maintained to provide safe and efficient staff/patient ratios. Staffing should be sufficient to provide assistance with preparation, procedure, recovery, ambulation, and transfer of the obese patient. For the benefit of the patient as well as the staff, education and development of systems for the safe transfer and mobilization of morbidly obese patients is imperative. It is the ideal to develop policies pertaining to these aspects and to conduct regular training sessions for education and quality improvement. Likewise, sensitivity training and training sessions in safe transfer and mobilization of obese patients should be included in the orientation of new staff that will have direct contact with bariatric patients.

Morbid obesity is associated with respiratory comorbidities including obstructive sleep apnea, restrictive lung disease, and pulmonary hypertension. During sedation, obese patients may develop alveolar hypoventilation. Sedation for bariatric patients undergoing endoscopic procedures is addressed in an article by John J. Vargo elsewhere in this issue. Access to anesthesia providers is apt to enhance proficiency. Individual sedation needs and risks may vary considerably among bariatric patients and endoscopic procedures. Ready access to experienced anesthesia providers, including certified registered nurse anesthetists, provides flexibility to respond to a greater number of circumstances.

ACLS training for physician and nursing staff is required. Ambulances servicing a free-standing endoscopy unit should also be equipped to manage bariatric patients with appropriate stretchers, straps, and transfer devices.

Summary

The battle against the epidemic of obesity is under way. For patients undergoing operative interventions, gastrointestinal endoscopy has a purpose in preoperative evaluation and the management of postoperative complications of bariatric surgery. Endoscopic bariatric procedures for weight loss are also emerging. Gastrointestinal endoscopy units will increasingly be expected to accommodate bariatric patients. Endoscopy unit considerations for the bariatric patient include access, space, facilities, equipment, staff and patient safety, and dignity. In addition to ordinary considerations, facilities catering for obese patients should comply with the standards of the Americans with Disabilities Act. Waiting rooms should be appointed to accommodate generously sized patients and their families. Doorways, hallways, and preparation and recovery spaces should be sized for passage of large-capacity rolling stretchers and wheelchairs. Staff must be experienced with and sensitive to the special needs of bariatric patients, and protected against ergonomic and lifting injuries. Specially rated procedure tables (stretchers) should be available for patients with class III obesity. Procedure-specific endoscopes and accessories should be available to perform endoscopic therapies unique to the bariatric patient population.

REFERENCES

1. SAGES Guidelines for office endoscopic services. (November 2008). Available at: http://www.sages.org/. Accessed January 8, 2011.
2. SAGES Guidelines for clinical application of laparoscopic bariatric surgery 2008. Available at: http://www.sages.org/. Accessed January 8, 2011.
3. ASMBS Bariatric Surgery Centers of Excellence Program. Available at: http://www.surgicalreview.org/COEPrograms/asmbs/hospitalprovisional.aspx; 2010 Surgical Review Corporation. Accessed January 8, 2011.
4. Pelczarski KM. Basic concerns in bariat. Healthc Des. March 2007. Available at: http://www.healthcaredesignmagazine.com. Accessed January 8, 2011.
5. Harrell JW, Miller B. Available at: http://www.hospitalconnect.com/hospitalconnect/index.jspBigchallenge: Designing for the needs of bariatric patients, March 15, 2004. Accessed January 8, 2011.
6. The American Institute of Architects. (2004). Planning and design guidelines for bariatric healthcare facilities. Available at: http://www.aia.org/nwsltr_print.cfm?

pagename=aah_jrnl_20061018_award_winner Created: Spring 2008. Accessed January 8, 2011.
7. American Society for Gastrointestinal Endoscopy: Establishment of gastrointestinal endoscopy areas. Gastrointest Endosc 1999;50:910–2.
8. Marasco JA, Marasco RF. Designing the ambulatory endoscopy center. Ambulatory Endoscopy Centers. Gastrointest Endosc Clin N Am 2002;12:185–204.
9. American Society for Gastrointestinal Endoscopy. Role of endoscopy in the bariatric surgery patient. Gastrointest Endosc 2008;68:1–10.

Endoscopic Management of Common Bariatric Surgical Complications

Jeanette N. Keith, MD[a,b,*]

KEYWORDS

• Endoscopic • Bariatric • Complications • Management

Bariatric procedures for the surgical treatment of obesity are increasing in number annually. In 2008, it is estimated that 220,000 procedures were performed in the United States by the membership of the American Society for Metabolic and Bariatric Surgery.[1] Although medical therapy is an effective intervention, weight loss surgery has been associated with the greatest reduction in obesity-related complications. With advances in technology and improved surgical techniques, the mortality following bariatric surgery is less than 1% at centers of excellence. Yet, approximately 5% to 10% of patients present for evaluation with acute postoperative complications[2] and 9% to 25% have late complications following bariatric surgery.[3] Early perioperative complications are defined as those that occur within the first 30 days of surgery, whereas late complications are those that occur after the first 30 days. The most common perioperative complications following bariatric surgery include anastomotic leaks, bowel obstruction, gastrointestinal or intra-abdominal hemorrhage, wound infection, deep vein thrombosis, and pulmonary embolus.[4] Complications such as anastomotic stricture, marginal ulcers (jejunal surface of the gastrojejunal anastomosis), gastric ulcers, stomal ulcers (gastric surface of the gastrojejunal anastomosis), bowel obstruction, incisional hernia, internal hernias, ischemia, nutrient deficiencies, hepatobiliary complications, band erosion, staple-line dehiscence, bile reflux, acid reflux, dumping syndrome, functional abdominal pain, and inadequate weight loss occur months to years following surgical weight loss interventions.[5–7] Whereas immediate symptoms in the first 30 days following surgery occasionally involve the

Financial disclosure: Research, A.S.P.E.N Rhoads Research Foundation, American Cancer Society, Dairy Management Incorporated; Consultant, NPS Pharmaceuticals; Speaker's Bureau, National Dairy Council; Stock Ownership (Spouse), CTK Clinical Consultants, LLC.

[a] Section of Gastroenterology, State University of New York, University of Buffalo, Buffalo, NY, USA

[b] Buffalo General Hospital, 100 High Street, Buffalo, NY 14203, USA

* Section of Gastroenterology, State University of New York, University of Buffalo, Buffalo, NY.

E-mail address: Jkeith2@buffalo.edu

Gastrointest Endoscopy Clin N Am 21 (2011) 275–285

doi:10.1016/j.giec.2011.02.007 giendo.theclinics.com

gastroenterologist, the primary role of nonsurgical endoscopic intervention postoperatively is in the management of late bariatric surgical complications and nonoperative revision of the surgical anatomy. In the future, indications for therapeutic endoscopy will undoubtedly expand the role of the gastroenterologist to include primary weight loss interventions, as the cutting-edge technology is currently undergoing rigorous scientific evaluation.[8] Therefore, endoscopists caring for these patients should become familiar with the post–bariatric surgical anatomy, potential complications, common presenting symptoms, anticipated luminal and extraluminal findings, and endoscopic management. This review discusses common presenting symptoms, luminal and extraluminal findings, and endoscopic management of common bariatric complications as outlined in **Table 1**.

PRESENTING SYMPTOMS AND ENDOSCOPIC FINDINGS

Several investigators report that 20% to 30% of bariatric surgical patients receiving care in academic medical centers and in community institutions present with symptoms that prompt endoscopic evaluation.[9,10] Huang and colleagues[9] found in 49 patients referred for evaluation following bariatric surgery that the major presenting symptoms were abdominal pain (53%), nausea with vomiting (35%), dysphagia (16%),

Table 1
Common bariatric complications: postsurgical endoscopic findings by procedure

Procedure Type	Restrictive	Restrictive	Restrictive	Malabsorptive	Combined	Combined
Procedure Name	GB	VBG	Sleeve	JIB	RYGB	DS
Complications:						
Band erosion	x	x				
Bezoar	x	x			x	
Disrupted staple/ sutures		x	x	x	x	x
Erosive esophagitis	x	x	x	x	x	x
Fistula		x	x	x	x	x
Food impaction	x	x			x	
Foreign material		x	x	x	x	x
Gallstones	x	x	x	x	x	x
Gastritis	x	x	x	x	x	x
GERD due to procedure	x	x	x			x
Leak		x	x	x	x	x
Stenosis/stricture		x	x	x	x	x
Ulcer, duodenal	x	x	x	x	x	x
Ulcer, gastric (pouch)	x	x	x	x	x	x
Ulcer, marginal (jejunal)		x			x	
Ulcer, stomal (gastric)		x			x	

Abbreviations: DS, sleeve gastrectomy with duodenal switch; GB, gastric band; GERD, gastroesophageal reflux disease; JIB, jejunoileal bypass; RYGB, Roux-en-Y gastric bypass; Sleeve, sleeve gastrectomy; VGB, vertical banded gastroplasty.

Courtesy of Jeanette N. Keith, Buffalo, NY.

gastrointestinal hemorrhage (12%), and weight regain (6%). Several patients had more than 1 symptom suggestive of a postsurgical complication, and the constellation of symptoms was predictive of endoscopic findings. When considering the predictive value of symptoms in 49 patients who underwent 69 procedures, the absence of nausea, vomiting, and dysphagia had a negative predictive value of 100% when assessing for the presence of stomal stenosis. Second, the time interval following surgery had a direct effect on the endoscopic findings. In the first 6 months following surgery, 85% of the endoscopies had at least 1 abnormal finding versus 47% after 6 months. Third, all symptomatic patients should be evaluated. Marano[10] found that, of 23 of 200 symptomatic bariatric surgical patients in a single community hospital, all complained of some degree of epigastric pain, nausea, and vomiting regardless of endoscopic findings. The most common findings were ulcer disease (52%), anastomotic stricture (4.3%), obstructed biliopancreatic limb (4.3%), acute gastric pouch bleed (4.3%), and anastomotic rupture/dehiscence (4.3%). Although 30% had normal postoperative anatomy and *Helicobacter pylori* infection was not detected in any patient in the population, uncommon complications must also be considered. In another large series, outcomes following 1292 consecutive divided Roux-en-Y gastric bypass surgeries were examined with approximately 17.6 months of follow-up.[11] Fifteen patients (1.2%) presented for endoscopic evaluation and were found to have gastrogastric fistulas. Of these, 12 (80%) complained of nausea, vomiting, and abdominal pain. Four patients (27%) presented because of failure to lose the expected amount of weight. On endoscopic examination, 8 patients (53%) were found to have a coexisting marginal ulcer, highlighting the need to consider the presence of a fistula or leak when an ulcer is found.

To evaluate the predictors of endoscopic findings, a retrospective review of 1001 bypass surgeries performed in an academic medical center was completed.[12] A total of 226 patients (166 open surgeries and 60 laparoscopic procedures), or 23% of the cohort, underwent endoscopic evaluation of gastrointestinal symptoms following surgery. Patients presented with nausea and vomiting (62%), abdominal pain (30%), dyspepsia (30%), early satiety (5%), dysphagia (4%), and heartburn (2%). Consistent with other series, the investigators found that 35% of the patients had more than 1 symptom. Other risk factors that were associated with a symptomatic presentation include nonsteroidal antiinflammatory drug (NSAID) use (27%), smoking (12%), and alcohol use (7%). About 14% were given proton pump inhibitor (PPI) therapy, and all had received 1 month of therapy with an H2 receptor antagonist for 1 month before surgery. On endoscopy, 127 patients had abnormal findings: marginal ulcer (36%), stomal stenosis (13%), and staple-line dehiscence (4%). Other less common findings (<3%) were esophagitis, nonmarginal ulcer, Schatzki ring, benign gastric polyps, and a solid food bezoar, with approximately 3% of the patients having more than 1 endoscopic finding. No gastrogastric fistulas were reported. Smoking, NSAID use, and abdominal pain predicted the presence of marginal ulcers at endoscopy; the use of PPI therapy was protective but only for the NSAID subgroup. Further, smoking and NSAID use predicted staple-line dehiscence. Age, gender, surgical technique, and surgeon experience did not predict abnormal findings at endoscopy. Time from surgery to presentation predicted findings for the presence of stomal ulcers and stomal stenosis. As in the series by Huang and colleagues,[9] presenting more than 6 months after surgery was associated with a lower likelihood of stomal ulceration or stenosis. In contrast, presenting after 6 months was associated with a greater likelihood of staple-line dehiscence.

In addition to indicating the possible presence of stomal ulceration or stenosis, abdominal pain following bariatric surgery may be reflective of symptomatic gallstones and hepatobiliary disease. Nearly 30% to 36% of patients undergoing any type of bariatric procedure develop gallstones generally within 6 months of surgery, with sludge developing in as many as 13% of patients.[13–15] Li and colleagues[16] found that weight loss of more than 25% of the original weight was an independent risk factor for the development of symptomatic gallstone formation. The management of asymptomatic gallstones and gallbladder disease before bariatric surgery remains debated.[17] Endoscopic therapy for symptomatic gallstones that develop in 4.7% to 7% of bariatric patients has also been described and is reviewed in the following section.

Symptoms associated with the nutritional complications of bariatric surgery are less specific and, thus, require a higher index of suspicion, as they coexist with abnormal endoscopic findings. Patients with persistent vomiting, rapid weight loss, or inadequate nutrient intake following any bariatric procedure are at risk for deficiencies such as thiamine deficiency.[18] Thiamine is a water-soluble vitamin that is not synthesized in vivo, requiring adequate dietary consumption. Dietary sources of thiamine include cereals, whole grains, lean pork, organ meat (liver), eggs, and legumes. Total depletion of the body's thiamine stores can occur within 20 days of surgery or in the setting of inadequate intake. If left untreated, thiamine deficiency can be fatal. Undertreatment or misdiagnosis can lead to preventable but irreversible clinical sequellae, including encephalopathy, paralysis, and heart failure.[19] Other nonspecific symptoms such as chronic diarrhea, muscle cramps, aplastic anemia, glossitis, unexplained weakness, or fatigue may be harbingers of underlying micronutrient deficiencies, indicating the need for small-bowel mucosal biopsies.[20] Further, other small-bowel mucosal disorders, such as celiac disease, may also be found in patients who present with nutritional deficiencies, including refractory iron deficiency anemia, after bariatric surgery.[21] Regardless of specialty, physicians caring for the post–bariatric surgical patients must be diligent to monitor for and treat nutritional deficiencies. Given the seriousness of this concern, the American Society for Metabolic and Bariatric Surgery, The Obesity Society, The Endocrine Society, the American Association of Clinical Endocrinologists, and the American Society for Parenteral and Enteral Nutrition have published guidelines for clinical practice that are worthy of review.[13,20] The upcoming bariatric guidelines from the American Gastroenterological Association and other leading gastrointestinal organizations should also be reviewed. The next section provides an overview of the most common complications that typically require endoscopic diagnosis or therapy. More detail is provided about the management of specific conditions in other articles in this issue.

ENDOSCOPIC MANAGEMENT OF COMMON BARIATRIC COMPLICATIONS

Stomal and Marginal Ulcers

Although bleeding duodenal ulcers have been rarely reported following Roux-en-Y gastric bypass,[22] ulcerations on the gastric side of the anastomosis (stomal ulcers) or on the jejunal surface of the anastomosis (marginal ulcers) occur in approximately 20% of patients. The cause of true stomal ulcers is thought to be ischemic in nature, whereas the cause of marginal ulcers is poorly understood.[23] Multiple mechanisms have been proposed to explain marginal ulcers. Local ischemia, larger pouch size leaving retained parietal cells that produce gastric acid, acidic gastric secretions poorly tolerated in the jejunum, NSAID use, alcohol use, smoking, a coexisting gastrogastric fistula, and the presence of a foreign body such as nonabsorbable suture material have been implicated.[24–27] The role of *H pylori* is not clear but has also been implicated as a risk factor in a review of 260 patients. *H pylori* serology may be the most reliable method for detecting the presence of the bacteria in this population, as pouch biopsies and breath tests may have problems with false-negative results. In patients who have been treated for *H pylori* infection, fecal antigen is a reliable method of detection.[28] In treating marginal ulcers, endoscopists are encouraged to remove nonabsorbable sutures when visible intraluminally to assist with healing, prevent gastrogastric fistulas, and relieve chronic abdominal pain in patients who underwent bariatric surgery.[29,30] Long-term treatment with oral Carafate and PPI therapy, along with antibiotics if *H pylori* infection is present, have led to healing of the ulcers. Refractory ulcers should raise concern for the presence of a gastrogastric fistula. In one study, marginal ulcer and associated gastrogastric fistula responded to a combination of PPI therapy and fibrin glue injections.[31] Healing times for ulcer resolution vary from 8 weeks to 6 months but were longer in the presence of an untreated or undiagnosed fistula.[5,8,27,32]

Stomal Stenosis

Stomal stenosis occurs in as many as 4.73% to 27% of patients undergoing Roux-en-Y gastric bypass.[33,34] These patients typically present with dysphagia, nausea with vomiting, or early satiety as previously noted. The primary endoscopic intervention is balloon dilation up to 15 to 18 mm, which has been associated with a greater than 93% success rate in symptom resolution and subsequent weight loss.[35,36] Dilation with Savary-Gilliard bougie (Cook Endoscopy; Winston-Salem, NC, USA) may be considered and is an effective intervention. In one review, both methods required 2 to 3 sessions of therapy, with a complication rate of 3%.[37] Gradual dilation over a few sessions is likely the best, as overdilation could potentially lead to loss of restriction and weight regain in some patients. For symptomatic patients presenting with refractory vomiting, thiamine repletion should be considered early and before exogenous glucose administration to prevent the precipitation of Wernicke encephalopathy.[38]

Gastrogastric Fistulas

Most large series report that gastrogastric fistulas occur in 1.2% to 1.8% of patients undergoing gastric bypass.[11,31] However, incidence rates from zero to as high as 46% have been reported, with substantial improvements in recent years because of modifications in the surgical technique.[39,40] Because of the high rate of morbidity and mortality associated with surgical revision of gastrogastric fistulas, initial treatment has evolved from surgical interventions to endoscopic management, with variable success. Reported endoscopic techniques include the use of fibrin glue sealants,[41,42] insertion of a Surgisis fistula plug (Cook Surgical, Inc, Bloomington, IN, USA) with or without a self-expanding stent,[43] endoluminal stent placement,[44] the use of mucosal suturing devices for tissue apposition,[45] and local debridement following argon plasma coagulation.[46] The optimal method of treatment is unknown, as comparison studies and randomized controlled trials are lacking.

Anastomotic Rupture/Dehiscence/Leaks

Published incidence rates for leaks following bariatric surgery range from 0.4% to 26%, and leaks are associated with a mortality rate of 1.5%.[47] Next to pulmonary embolus, intra-abdominal sepsis secondary to leaks is the most serious life-threatening complication associated with bariatric surgery. The potential causes of leaks are multiple: tension on the anastomosis, staple or stapler malfunction, suture or staple-line seepage, poor surgical technique, obstruction, hypovascularization, and hematomas.[48] Leaks require early recognition of symptoms, detection, and prompt treatment to prevent loss of life. Recent reports demonstrate that endoluminal interventions are effective in healing anastomotic breeches. Multiple investigators are reporting the successful placement of covered endoluminal stents and the initiation of oral nutrition leading to recovery from this postoperative complication.[49–51] Nonsurgical interventions were found to result in the healing of anastomotic leaks in 17 of 21, or 81%, of affected patients.[52]

Hepatobiliary Complications Including Cholelithiasis

The development of hepatobiliary disease is common following bariatric surgery.[53] Shiffman and colleagues[15] reported that gallstones developed in 36% and sludge developed in 13% of 81 patients with normal gallbladder ultrasonograms at the time of surgery. About 40% of these subjects developed symptoms, and 28% underwent elective cholecystectomy. Controversies exist as to the best evaluation and treatment of this high-risk population. At present, only 30% of surgeons actively perform elective preoperative cholecystectomy procedures to remove normal-appearing gallbladders.[54] Although prophylactic administration of ursodiol has decreased the frequency of gallstone disease requiring intervention to 2%, it is not widely prescribed. In fact, some practitioners have questioned the validity of prophylactic management.[55,56]

Because the incidence of hepatobiliary complications is high, evaluation should be performed in a systematic fashion to identify those who need endoscopic intervention. To evaluate a symptomatic patient for the presence of stones or other hepatobiliary disease, magnetic resonance imaging (MRI) or computed tomography (CT) is preferred, as ultrasound image resolution is adversely affected by body fat, contributing to missed diagnoses.[57] When symptomatic disease occurs, endoscopic retrograde cholangiopancreatography is the gold standard procedure for nonsurgical therapeutic management of hepatobiliary disease. The endoscopic approach is complicated by the post–bariatric surgical anatomy, limiting transoral access. Laparoscopy-assisted transgastric approach is the most commonly reported intervention.[58,59] Single-balloon[60] and double-balloon[61] enteroscopy and temporary restoration of digestive continuity have been advocated, allowing for stone extraction and sphincterotomy as indicated.[62]

Weight Regain

Although highly debated, it has been reported that 18% to 30% of bariatric patients experience a near-total weight regain following bariatric surgery, constituting surgical failure.[63,64] Although weight regain or failure to lose weight following a bariatric procedure is typically considered to be related to dietary indiscretions, failure to exercise,[65] or failure of the body to maintain the surgically induced changes in regulatory gut hormones such as peptide YY,[66] other causes that are amenable to endoscopic intervention have been identified. Loss of restriction because of a dilated gastrojejunostomy and/or a dilated gastric pouch after bariatric surgery results in weight gain as a consequence of loss of satiation and increased caloric intake. Some investigators point out that stomal size correlates with the risk of weight regain for bariatric patients.[67] Therefore, when patients present with weight regain or failure to lose weight, endoscopic evaluation and radiologic studies should be considered.[68] When an enlarged gastrojejunal stoma is found, potential endoscopic interventions that promote restriction and facilitate additional weight loss include (1) sclerotherapy of the site using 6 to 30 mL of sodium morrhuate injected circumferentially, which is associated with a 72% to 75% success rate[69–73]; (2) the use of a tissue plication system to reduce the size of the gastrojejunostomy and the gastric pouch, known as the revision obesity surgery endoscopic procedure;[74–76] (3) revisional surgery using a tissue plication device known as StomaPhyX (EndoGatric Solutions; Redwood City, CA, USA) to reduce the pouch size;[77] and (4) application of the endoclip to reduce the size of the gastrojejunal anastomosis.[78] Weight regain may also indicate the presence of a gastrogastric fistula, which may be addressed endoscopically in a similar manner.[11] Although endoscopic therapy facilitates weight loss, it must be accompanied by dietary, behavioral, and lifestyle changes to ensure long-term success.

SUMMARY

Obesity is a major public health concern affecting 32.2% of adult men and 35.5% of adult women in the United States.[79] As more patients undergo bariatric surgery, the need for the practicing gastroenterologists to recognize and treat early and late complications of weight loss surgical procedures is increasing and will undoubtedly become the standard of care for comprehensive weight loss centers that care for these patients. Although this review addresses the most common bariatric complications, clinicians are encouraged to seek advanced training that will help them to identify these complications and develop proficiency in performing the advanced procedures to treat them. As new procedures emerge and additional potential complications are identified, institutions should actively develop protocols to manage this high-risk patient population.[20]

REFERENCES

1. Metabolic and Bariatric Surgery Fact Sheet. The American Society for Metabolic and Bariatric Surgery. Available at: http://www.asbs.org/Newsite07/media/asmbs_fs_surgery.pdf. Accessed December 15, 2010.
2. Pories WJ. Bariatric surgery: risks and rewards. J Clin Endocrinol Metab 2008;93:S89–96.
3. Parikh MS, Laker S, Weiner M, et al. Objective comparison of complications resulting from laparoscopic bariatric procedures. J Am Coll Surg 2006;202:252–61.
4. Herron DM, Bloomberg R. Complications of bariatric surgery. Minerva Chir 2006;6:125–39.
5. Nguyen NT, Wilson SE. Complications of antiobesity surgery. Nat Clin Pract Gastroenterol Hepatol 2007;4:138–47.
6. Decker GA, Swain JM, Crowell MD, et al. Gastrointestinal and nutritional complications after bariatric surgery. Am J Gastroenterol 2007;102:2571–80.
7. Monkhouse SJ, Morgan JD, Norton SA. Complications of bariatric surgery: presentation and emergency management–a review. Ann R Coll Surg Engl 2009;91:280–6.
8. Schauer P, Chand B, Brethauer S. New applications for endoscopy: the emerging field of endoluminal and transgastric bariatric surgery. Surg Endosc 2007;21:347–56.
9. Huang CS, Forse RA, Jacobsen BC, et al. Endoscopic findings and their clinical correlation in patients with symptoms after gastric bypass surgery. Gastrointest Endosc 2003;58:859–66.
10. Marano BJ Jr. Endoscopy after Roux-en Y gastric bypass: a community hospital experience. Obes Surg 2005;15:342–5.
11. Carrodeguas L, Szomstein S, Soto F, et al. Management of gastrogastric fistulas after divided Roux-en Y gastric bypass surgery for morbid obesity: analysis of 1,292 consecutive patients and review of the literature. Surg Obes Relat Dis 2005;1:467–74.

12. Wilson JA, Romagnuolo J, Byrne TK, et al. Predictors of endoscopic findings after Roux-en Y gastric bypass. Am J Gastroenterol 2006;101:2194–9.
13. Mechanick JI, Kushner RF, Sugerman HJ, et al. American Society of Clinical Endocrinologists, The Obesity Society and American Society for Metabolic and Bariatric Surgery medical guidelines for the clinical practice for the perioperative, metabolic and nonsurgical support of the bariatric surgery patient. Obesity (Silver Spring) 2009;17:1–70.
14. Iglezias Brandao de Oliveira C, Adami Chaim E, Borges da Silva B. Impact of rapid weight reduction on risk of cholelithiasis after bariatric surgery. Obes Surg 2003;13:625–8.
15. Shiffman ML, Sugerman HJ, Kellum JM, et al. Gallstone formation after rapid weight loss: a prospective study in patients undergoing gastric bypass surgery for treatment of morbid obesity. Am J Gastroenterol 1991;86:1000–5.
16. Li VK, Pulido N, Fajnwaks P, et al. Predictors of gallstone formation after bariatric surgery: a multivariate analysis of risk factors comparing gastric bypass, gastric banding and sleeve gastrectomy. Surg Endosc 2009;23:1640–4.
17. Patel JA, Patel NA, Smith DE 3rd, et al. Perioperative management of cholelithiasis in patients presenting for laparoscopic Roux-en Y gastric bypass: have we reached a consensus? Am Surg 2009;75:470–6.
18. Shankar P, Boylan M, Sriram K. Micronutrient deficiencies after bariatric surgery. Nutrition 2010;26:1031–7.
19. Aasheim ET. Wernicke encephalopathy after bariatric surgery—a systematic review. Ann Surg 2008;248:714–20.
20. Heber D, Greenway FL, Kaplan LM, et al. Endocrine and nutritional management of the post-bariatric surgery patient: an endocrine society practice guideline. J Clin Endocrinol Metab 2010;95:4823–43.
21. Gisbert JP, Gomolion F. A short review of malabsorption and anemia. World J Gastroenterol 2009;15:4644–52.
22. Mittermair R, Renz O. An unusual complication of gastric bypass: perforated duodenal ulcer. Obes Surg 2007;17:701–3.
23. Dallal RM, Bailey LA. Ulcer diseases after gastric bypass surgery. Surg Obes Relat Dis 2006;2:455–9.
24. Garrido AB Jr, Rossi M, Lima SE Jr, et al. Early marginal ulcer following Roux-en-Y gastric bypass under proton pump inhibitor treatment: prospective multicentric study. Arq Gastroenterol 2010;47:130–4.
25. Yu S, Jastrow K, Clapp B, et al. Foreign material erosion after laparoscopic Roux-en Y gastric bypass: findings and treatment. Surg Endosc 2007;21:1216–20.
26. Csendes A, Burgos AM, Altuve J, et al. Incidence of marginal ulcer 1 month and 1 to 2 years after gastric bypass: a prospective consecutive endoscopic evaluation of 442 patients with morbid obesity. Obes Surg 2009;19:135–8.
27. Gumbs AA, Duffy AJ, Bell RL. Incidence and management of marginal ulceration after laparoscopic Roux-en Y gastric bypass. Surg Obes Relat Dis 2006;2:460–3.
28. Rasmussen JJ, Fuller W, Ali MR. Marginal ulceration after laparoscopic gastric bypass: an analysis of predisposing factors in 260 patients. Surg Endosc 2007;21:1090–4.
29. Frezza EE, Herbert H, Ford R, et al. Endoscopic suture removal at gastrojejunal anastomosis after Roux-en Y gastric bypass to prevent marginal ulceration. Surg Obes Relat Dis 2007;3:619–22.
30. Ryou M, Mogobgab O, Lautz DB, et al. Endoscopic foreign body removal for treatment of chronic abdominal pain in patients after Roux-en-Y gastric bypass. Surg Obes Relat Dis 2010;6:526–31.

31. Gumbs AA, Duffy AJ, Bell RL. Management of gastrogastric fistula after laparoscopic Roux-en Y gastric bypass. Surg Obes Relat Dis 2006;2:117–21.
32. Schirmer BD. Stricture and marginal ulcers in bariatric surgery. In: Buchwald H, Cowan GS, Pories W, editors. Surgical management of obesity. Philadelphia: WB Saunders; 2006. p. 297–303.
33. Podnos YD, Jimenez JC, Wilson SE, et al. Complications after laparoscopic gastric bypass. Arch Surg 2003;138:957–61.
34. Matthews BD, Sing RF, Delegge MH, et al. Initial results with a stapled gastrojejunostomy for the laparoscopic isolated Roux-en Y gastric bypass. Am J Surg 2000;179:476–81.
35. Peifer KJ, Shiels AJ, Azar R, et al. Successful endoscopic management of gastrojejunal anastomotic strictures after Roux-en Y gastric bypass. Gastrointest Endosc 2007;66:248–52.
36. Ukleja A, Afonso BB, Pimental R, et al. Outcome of endoscopic balloon dilation of strictures after laparoscopic gastric bypass. Surg Endosc 2008;22: 1746–50.
37. Ellsmere JC, Thompson CC, Brugge WR, et al. Endoscopic interventions for weight loss surgery. Obesity (Silver Spring) 2009;17:929–33.
38. Boxbora A, Coskun H, Ozarmagan S, et al. A rare complication of adjustable gastric banding: Wernicke's encephalopathy. Obes Surg 2000;10:274–5.
39. Filho AJ, Kondo W, Nassif LS, et al. Gastrogastric fistula: a possible complication of Roux-en Y gastric bypass. JSLS 2006;10:326–31.
40. Cucchi SG, Pories WJ, MacDonald KG, et al. Gastrogastric fistulas: a complication of divided gastric bypass surgery. Ann Surg 1995;221:387–91.
41. Papayramidis ST, Eleftheriadis EE, Papayramidis TS, et al. Endoscopic management of gastrocutaneous fistula after bariatric surgery by using a fibrin sealant. Gatrointest Endosc 2004;59:296–300.
42. Papayramidis TS, Kotzampassi K, Kotidis E, et al. Endoscopic fibrin sealing of gastrocutaneous fistula after sleeve gastrectomy and biliopancreatic diversion with duodenal switch. J Gastroenterol Hepatol 2008;23:1802–5.
43. Toussaint E, Eisendrath P, Kwan V, et al. Endoscopic treatment of postoperative enterocutaneous fistulas after surgery with the use of a fistula plug: report of five cases. Endoscopy 2009;41:560–3.
44. Eisendrath P, Cremer M, Himpens J, et al. Endotherapy including temporary stenting of fistulas of the upper gastrointestinal tract after laparoscopic bariatric surgery. Endoscopy 2007;39:625–30.
45. Fernandez-Esparrach G, Lautz DB, Thompson CC. Endoscopic repair of gastrogastric fistula after Roux-en-Y gastric bypass: a less-invasive approach. Surg Obes Relat Dis 2010;6:282–8.
46. Bhardwaj A, Cooney RN, Wehrman A, et al. Endoscopic repair of small symptomatic gastrogastric fistulas after gastric bypass surgery: a single center experience. Obes Surg 2010;20:1090–5.
47. Fox SR, Srikanth MS. Leaks and gastric disruption in bariatric surgery. In: Buchwald H, Cowan GS, Pories WJ, editors. Surgical management of obesity. Philadelphia: WB Saunders; 2006. p. P304–12.
48. Fernandez AZ. Experience with over 3000 open and laparoscopic bariatric procedures: multivariate analysis of factors related to leak and resultant mortality. Surg Endosc 2004;18:193–7.
49. Eubanks S, Edwards CA, Fearing NM, et al. Use of endoscopic stents to treat anastomotic complications after bariatric surgery. J Am Coll Surg 2008;206: 935–9.

50. Serra C, Baltasar A, Andreo L, et al. Treatment of gastric leaks with coated self-expanding stents after sleeve gastrectomy. Obes Surg 2007;17:866–72.
51. Barbor R, Talbot M, Tyndal A. Treatment of upper gastrointestinal leaks with a removable, covered, self-expanding metallic stent. Surg Laparosc Endosc Percutan Tech 2009;19:e1–4.
52. Salinas A, Baptista A, Santiago E, et al. Self-expandable metal stents to treat gastric leaks. Surg Obes Relat Dis 2006;2:570–2.
53. Jonas E, Marsk R, Rasmussen F, et al. Incidence of postoperative gallstone disease after antiobesity surgery: population-based study from Sweden. Surg Obes Relat Dis 2010;6:54–8.
54. Mason EE, Renquist KE. Gallbladder management in obesity surgery. Obes Surg 2002;12:222–9.
55. Sugerman HJ, Brewer WH, Shiffman ML, et al. A multicenter, placebo-controlled, randomized, double-blind, prospective trial of prophylactic ursodiol for the prevention of gallstone formation following gastric-bypass-induced rapid weight loss. Am J Surg 1995;169:91–6.
56. Caruana JA, McCabe NM, Smith AD, et al. Incidence of symptomatic gallstones after gastric bypass: is prophylactic treatment really necessary? Surg Obes Relat Dis 2005;1:564–7.
57. Fiegler W, Felix R, Langer M, et al. Fat as a factor affecting resolution in diagnostic ultrasound: possibilities for improving picture quality. Eur J Radiol 1985;5:304–9.
58. Patel JA, Patel NA, Shinde T, et al. Endoscopic retrograde cholangiopancreatography after laparoscopic Roux-en-Y gastric bypass: a case series and review of the literature. Am Surg 2008;74:689–94.
59. Gutierrez JM, Lederer H, Krook JC, et al. Surgical gastrostomy for pancreatobiliary and duodenal access following Roux-en-Y gastric bypass. J Gastrointest Surg 2009;13:2170–5.
60. Wang A, Sauer BG, Behm BW, et al. Single-balloon enteroscopy effectively enables diagnostic and therapeutic retrograde cholangiography in patients with surgically altered anatomy. Gastrointest Endosc 2010;71:641–9.
61. Moreels TG, Huben GJ, Ysebaert DK, et al. Diagnostic and therapeutic double-balloon enteroscopy after small bowel reconstructive Roux-en-Y reconstructive surgery. Digestion 2009;80:141–7.
62. Saget A, Facchiano E, Bosset PO, et al. Temporary restoration of digestive continuity after laparoscopic bypass to allow endoscopic sphincterotomy and retrograde exploration of the biliary tract. Obes Surg 2010;20:791–5.
63. Magro DO, Geloneze B, Delfini R, et al. Long-term weight regain after gastric bypass: a 5 year prospective study. Obes Surg 2008;18:648–51.
64. Karmali S, Stoklossa CJ, Sharma A, et al. Bariatric surgery: a primer. Can Fam Physician 2010;56:873–9.
65. Kofman MD, Lent MR, Swencionis C. Maladaptive eating patterns, quality of life and weight outcomes following gastric bypass: result of an internet survey. Obesity (Silver Spring) 2010;18:1938–43.
66. Mequid MM, Glade MJ, Middleton FA. Weight regain after Roux-en-Y: a significant 20% complication related to PYY. Nutrition 2008;24:832–42.
67. Davveh BK, Lautz DB, Thompson CC. Gastrojejunal stoma diameter predicts weight regain after Roux-en Y gastric bypass. Clin Gastroenterol Hepatol 2010. [Epub ahead of print].
68. Brethauer SA, Nfonsam V, Sherman V, et al. Endoscopy and upper gastrointestinal contrast studies are complementary in evaluation of weight regain after bariatric surgery. Surg Obes Relat Dis 2006;2:643–50.

69. Spaulding L, Osler T, Patlak J. Long-term results of sclerotherapy for dilated gastrojejunostomy after gastric bypass. Surg Obes Relat Dis 2007;3:623–6.
70. Catalano MF, Rudic G, Anderson AJ, et al. Weight gain after bariatric surgery as a result of a large gastric stoma: endotherapy with sodium morrhuate may prevent the need for surgical revision. Gastrointest Endosc 2007;66:240–5.
71. Madan AK, Martiniz JM, Khan KA, et al. Endoscopic sclerotherapy for dilated gastrojejunostomy after gastric bypass. J Laparoendosc Adv Surg Tech A 2010;20:235–7.
72. Spaulding L. Treatment of dilated gastrojejunostomy with sclerotherapy. Obes Surg 2003;13:254–7.
73. Loewen M, Barba C. Endoscopic sclerotherapy for dilated gastrojejunostomy of failed gastric bypass. Surg Obes Relat Dis 2008;4:539–43.
74. Ryou M, Mullady DK, Lautz DB, et al. Pilot study evaluating technical feasibility and early outcomes of a second-generation endosurgical platform for treatment of weight regain after gastric bypass surgery. Surg Obes Relat Dis 2009;5:450–4.
75. Mullady DK, Lautz DB, Thompson CC. Treatment of weight regain after gastric bypass surgery when using a new endoscopic platform: initial experience and early outcomes (with video). Gastrointest Endosc 2009;70:440–4.
76. Thompson CC, Slattery J, Bundga ME, et al. Peroral endoscopic reduction of dilated gastrojejunal anastomosis after Roux-en-Y gastric bypass: a possible new option for patients with weight regain. Surg Endosc 2006;20:1744–8.
77. Mikami D, Needleman B, Narula V, et al. Natural orifice surgery: initial US experience utilizing the StomaphyX device to reduce gastric pouches after Roux-en-Y gastric bypass. Surg Endosc 2010;24:223–8.
78. Hylen AM, Jacobs A, Lybeer M, et al. The OTSC-clip in revisional endoscopy against weight gain after bariatric gastric bypass surgery. Obes Surg 2010. [Epub ahead of print].
79. Flegal KM, Carroll MD, Ogden CL, et al. Prevalence and trends in obesity among US adults, 1999–2008. JAMA 2010;303:235–41.

Management of Acute Postoperative Hemorrhage in the Bariatric Patient

Lincoln E.V.V. Ferreira, MD, PhD[a], Louis M. Wong Kee Song, MD[b], Todd H. Baron, MD[b,*]

KEYWORDS

- Gastrointestinal bleeding • Endoscopic treatment • Obesity
- Bariatric surgery • Postoperative hemorrhage
- Post-bariatric bleeding

Bariatric surgery is one of the treatment options to achieving and preserving weight loss and to managing medical complications related to obesity. With the obesity epidemic, the number of bariatric procedures performed annually has risen exponentially over the past two decades.[1–3] In the United States, laparoscopic Roux-en-Y gastric bypass (LRYGB) has become the gold standard procedure for morbid obesity. After bariatric surgery, early or late adverse events can occur. Although bariatric surgery is considered safe, especially with the advent of laparoscopic techniques, complications still occur. Systemic complications include malnutrition and vitamin deficiencies, thromboembolism, and infection. Local complications include anastomotic leaks and strictures, fistulas, marginal ulcers, staple line disruption, band erosion, small bowel obstruction, incisional or internal hernias, and intraluminal or extraluminal gastrointestinal (GI) hemorrhage.[2]

The approach to early postoperative GI hemorrhage (arbitrarily defined as bleeding occurring within 2 weeks after bariatric surgery) differs from that of bleeding in patients with native gut anatomy. Early GI bleeding is more often a complication associated with Roux-en-Y gastric bypass (RYGB) surgery than other bariatric procedures and usually involves the gastrojejunostomy anastomosis. GI bleeding that occurs beyond the early postoperative period commonly involves the staple line at the gastrojejunal or

Dr LEVV Ferreira has nothing to disclose.

[a] Department of Medicine, Digestive Endoscopy Unit, Hospital Universitario da Universidade Federal de Juiz de Fora, Unidade de Endoscopia Digestiva-Avenida Eugenio do Nascimento s/nº. Bairro: Dom Bosco – CEP:36038-330, Juiz de Fora, Minas Gerais, Brasil
[b] Mayo GI Bleeding Team, Division of Gastroenterology and Hepatology, Mayo Clinic, 200 First Street SW, Rochester, MN 55905, USA
* Corresponding author.
E-mail address: baron.todd@mayo.edu

Gastrointest Endoscopy Clin N Am 21 (2011) 287–294
doi:10.1016/j.giec.2011.02.002 giendo.theclinics.com
1052-5157/11/$ – see front matter

jejunojejunal anastomotic sites (marginal ulcers) or bypassed stomach. This review focuses on the current status and management of early GI bleeding after bariatric surgery.

EPIDEMIOLOGY

Early postoperative bleeding occurs in 1% to 5% of cases after RYGB.[3–5] The variable reported rates for early bleeding depend on the definition used for "early" hemorrhage, type of surgery performed (laparoscopic vs open), type of bleeding described (eg, intraluminal or extraluminal), perioperative use of antithrombotic agents, and threshold used to differentiate bleeding from normal postoperative hemodilution.

In a meta-analysis involving 3464 RYGB patients, the reported rate for acute postoperative GI bleeding was 1.9%.[3] In another study, early postoperative hemorrhage occurred in 33 of 1025 patients (3.2%) who underwent RYGB; bleeding was extraluminal in almost 50% of cases.[4] Similar to other study findings, the postoperative bleeding rate was higher in the laparoscopic group than in the open group (5.1% vs 2.4%). Rebleeding episodes may also occur more commonly in this patient population. In a retrospective study involving 933 LRYGB patients, 30 (3.2%) developed acute postoperative bleeding. Of these, a single bleeding episode occurred in 14 (47%) patients; two bleeding episodes occurred in 13 (43%) patients; and three bleeding episodes occurred in 3 (10%) patients.[5] In another study of 518 patients who underwent LRYGB, the rate of early postoperative bleeding was 3.9%; 80% of the bleeding was extraluminal and 20% was intraluminal.[6]

Postoperative bleeding is a rare complication after vertical banded gastroplasty, laparoscopic adjustable gastric banding, and laparoscopic sleeve gastrectomy.[7–10] Death after bariatric surgery as a consequence of acute bleeding is uncommon. In a retrospective study of 13,871 patients who underwent bariatric surgery, 34 deaths were reported. Of these, only one was due to a bleeding gastric ulcer after biliopancreatic diversion.[11]

PREDISPOSING FACTORS

Obesity itself is an independent risk factor for venous thromboembolism.[12–14] The risk for a thromboembolic event, including deep vein thrombosis and pulmonary embolism, is increased further in patients undergoing bariatric surgery.[14] Because the risk may be as high as 3.1%, several measures are implemented to reduce the rate of postoperative venous thromboembolism, including early ambulation, compression stockings, and administration of prophylactic heparin.[15–19] Drugs, such as heparin and clopidogrel, have been used to prevent thromboembolic events but the risk of postoperative bleeding using these agents must be balanced against the risk of postoperative thromboembolic events.[20,21]

In a retrospective study, no correlation was seen between serum levels of anti-Xa and use of low molecular weight heparin (LMWH) and the risk of postoperative bleeding.[22] In contrast, another retrospective study demonstrated an increased incidence of early hemorrhage after RYGB in patients who received preoperative LMWH.[4] In patients receiving prophylactic antithrombotic agents after LRYGB, unfractionated heparin was associated with a lower incidence of acute postoperative bleeding than enoxaparin.[20] In a recent prospective study, an extended 3-week LMWH protocol was used for prophylaxis of venous thromboembolism in 735 patients who underwent laparoscopic bariatric surgery. The incidence of postoperative venous thromboembolism was 0% and only 3 adverse bleeding events occurred.[23] In the presence of clinically overt GI bleeding, the administration of heparin products should be discontinued.

Limited data are available regarding the risk for early postoperative GI bleeding associated with the use of antiplatelet agents, such as clopidogrel. One study reported patients undergoing gastric bypass having a high bleeding rate while taking clopidogrel, but all bleeding cases were late events occurring at 25 to 234 days from surgery.[21]

Ketorolac, an injectable nonsteroidal anti-inflammatory drug with strong antiplatelet activity, is often used as an alternative to opioid analgesia for relief of postsurgical pain.[24] After a single dose of ketorolac, platelet aggregation is disturbed for at least 24 hours.[25] In one study, however, no correlation was seen between the use of ketorolac and perioperative bleeding in postbariatric surgery patients despite the concomitant use of heparin.[4]

DIAGNOSIS AND INITIAL MANAGEMENT

The majority of GI bleeding occurs in the intraoperative or immediate postoperative period.[26,27] In one study, 70% of bleeding cases manifested themselves within 4 hours after surgery.[6] Early GI bleeding may be intraluminal or extraluminal. When extraluminal, an increase in abdominal drain output of blood becomes an essential indicator of postoperative bleeding and allows bleeding to be recognized early so that prophylactic anticoagulants can be discontinued.[28,29] In addition, based on the drainage output, it is possible to determine the rate of extraluminal bleeding and the need for transfusion and re-exploration.[28] When blood clots occlude the drain, however, when kinking of the drain occurs, or when incorrectly positioned, extraluminal bleeding may not be recognized.[6] Alternatively, the diagnosis of intraluminal hemorrhage is readily apparent in the presence of hematemesis, melena, or hematochezia. Associated symptoms and signs of bleeding may include tachycardia, hypotension, drop in hemoglobin, and even small bowel obstruction from blood clots. Extraluminal (intra-abdominal) hemorrhage occurs in as many as half of early postoperative bleeding cases and requires a high index of suspicion because cardinal signs of GI bleeding (eg, melena) are absent.[4] Patients complaining of more abdominal pain than expected and those with diffuse abdominal tenderness with hypoactive bowel sounds and a pattern of cyclic tachycardia (100 to 120 beats per minute) should be considered to have postsurgical bleeding even in the absence of an increase in abdominal drain output.[6]

Obtaining an abdominal imaging study (eg, CT scan) should be considered, particularly when alarm symptoms, such as tachycardia, oliguria, abdominal distention, and a precipitous fall in hematocrit, are present.[4]

In most patients, early postoperative GI bleeding is mild and can be managed conservatively, including the withholding of antithrombotic agents. Some investigators suggest that diagnostic studies are unnecessary, because the source of bleeding is more likely at the staple line.[4,17] In a review that included 89 GI bleeding cases after LRYGB, clinical observation alone was sufficient in 18 (20%); 49 patients (55%) required only fluid replacement and blood transfusion. Surgery was necessary in 18 (20%) patients who were hemodynamically unstable or remained unstable with ongoing bleeding despite fluid and blood transfusion.[25] In another study, 7/20 patients (35%) required surgical intervention to manage bleeding.[6]

THE ROLE OF ENDOSCOPY IN EARLY POSTOPERATIVE HEMORRHAGE

Endoscopic management of early postoperative intraluminal bleeding is challenging and controversial due to the risk of dehiscence and perforation at the surgical

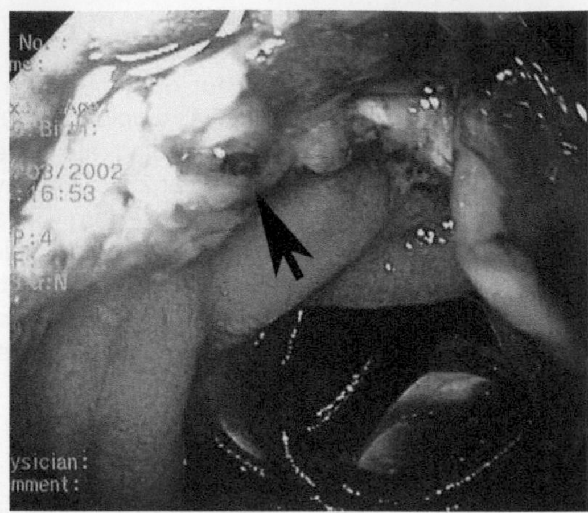

Fig. 1. Endoscopic view of gastrojejunal anastomosis of RYGB patient who developed overt GI bleeding on the second postoperative day. A visible vessel (*arrow*) is seen.

anastomosis.[4,17,30,31] Endoscopy is usually not necessary because bleeding is mild and self-limited in most cases but should be considered in patients in whom bleeding is severe (hemodynamic instability and/or ≥2 g drop in hemoglobin) or when rebleeding occurs after conservative management. If endoscopy is performed, air insufflation should be minimized to prevent disruption of the anastomosis and close communication with the surgeon is essential.

Early postoperative bleeding in RYGB most likely originates at the gastrojejunostomy and should be within reach of a standard upper endoscope (**Figs. 1** and **2**). On occasion, postoperative nausea and vomiting may lead to a bleeding Mallory-Weiss tear, which can be readily managed endoscopically.[32] In rare circumstances, bleeding occurs at the jejunojejunostomy or in the excluded stomach (eg, stress ulcers). Push enteroscopy or, preferably, balloon-assisted enteroscopy[33] may be

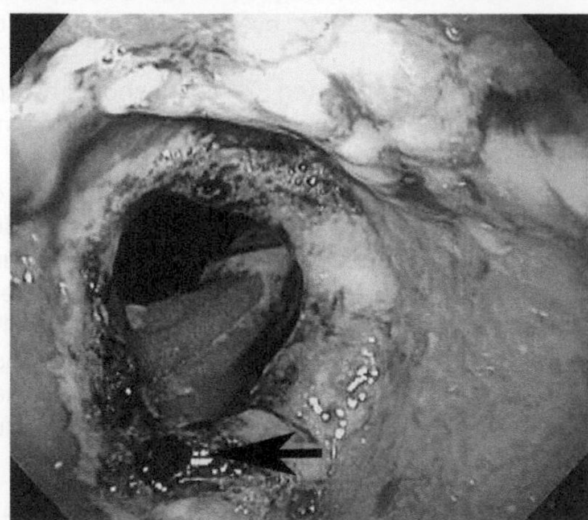

Fig. 2. Endoscopic view of gastrojejunal anastomosis of RYGB patient who developed overt GI bleeding on the first postoperative day. Multiple flat pigmented spots and adherent clot (*arrow*) are seen.

considered in these situations but extreme caution is warranted during the performance of enteroscopy in the early postoperative period because excessive gut stretching during push endoscopy or undue tension during pleating of the small bowel onto the overtube during balloon-assisted enteroscopy may result in anastomotic disruption. Alternatively, laparoscopic-assisted or laparotomy-assisted endoscopy can be performed (**Fig. 3**).

Studies addressing the role of endoscopy in postbariatric patients with early GI bleeding are limited.[5,26,34–37] In a review of 89 patients with acute perioperative bleeding after LRYGB, 77% of the patients could be treated without the need for endoscopic, radiologic, or surgical intervention. Diagnostic and therapeutic endoscopy was used in only 6 (6.7%) and 5 (5.6%) of these patients, respectively.[26] In contrast, Jamil and colleagues[5] proceeded with upper endoscopy in 27 of 30 patients (90%) with postoperative bleeding after LRYGB, and the source of bleeding was from the gastrojejunal anastomosis in all patients. Most patients (20/27; 74%) underwent endoscopy in an operating room and were endotracheally intubated (19/27; 70%). Bleeding stigmata seen at the gastrojejunostomy included active oozing (48%), visible

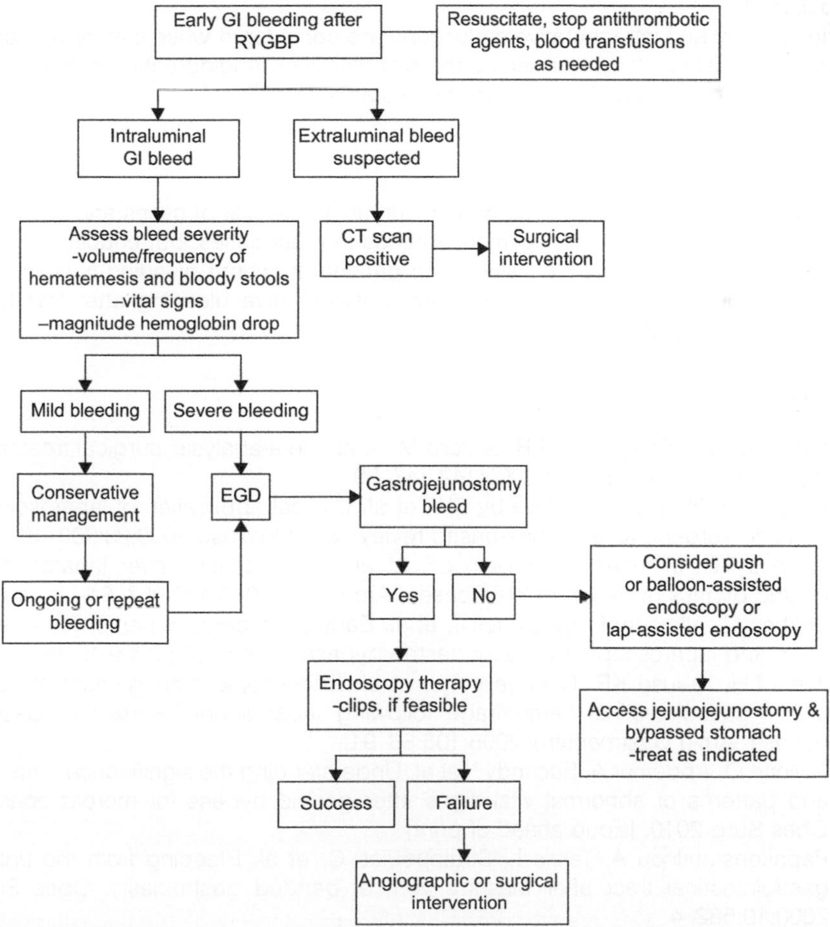

Fig. 3. Proposed management algorithm for early GI hemorrhage after RYGB surgery.

vessel (26%), and adherent clot (26%). Endoscopic therapy was performed in 85% of patients and included epinephrine injection, heater probe coagulation, combination epinephrine injection and thermal coagulation, and hemoclip placement in 3 (13%), 4 (17%), 14 (61%), and 2 (9%) patients, respectively. Initial hemostasis was achieved in all patients, but 5 (17%) patients required repeat endoscopy with therapy for rebleeding. None of the patients required surgery to control hemorrhage but two complications occurred (pulmonary aspiration and perforation).[5]

In patients in whom endoscopic therapy is considered, the use of endoclips is preferred, when technically feasible. Unlike sclerosant injection and thermal coagulation, endoscopic clips do not produce additional tissue injury and can be used to manage concomitant anastomotic leaks and iatrogenic perforations.[34] Three types of endoclips are commercially available: QuickClip2 Long, 11 mm when fully opened (Olympus America, Center Valley, PA, USA); TriClip, 3 prongs in a tripod configuration, 12 mm when opened (Cook Endoscopy, Winston-Salem, NC, USA); and Resolution Clip, 12 mm when fully opened (Boston Scientific, Natick, MA, USA). Clinical comparative data between the various clips are lacking; however, in an experimental animal study of acute ulcers, the initial rate of hemostasis was similar for all 3 clips. The clip retention rate was significantly higher with the Resolution Clip than the other 2 endoclips.[38]

Angiography and intraoperative endoscopy are considered when standard endoscopy fails to detect, reach, or secure the bleeding site. Angiographic embolization, however, can potentially devascularize fresh staple lines.[26]

SUMMARY

Early GI bleeding after bariatric surgery occurs in 1% to 5% of cases and is usually self-limited. Conservative management suffices in most cases, but endoscopy with therapeutic intent should be considered in patients in whom bleeding is severe or recurs. A management algorithm for early postoperative bleeding after RYGB is proposed (see **Fig. 3**).

REFERENCES

1. Maggard MA, Shugarman LR, Suttorp M, et al. Meta-analysis: surgical treatment of obesity. Ann Intern Med 2005;142:547–59.
2. Farrell TM, Haggerty SP, Overby DW, et al. Clinical application of laparoscopic bariatric surgery: an evidence-based review. Surg Endosc 2009;23:930–49.
3. Podnos YD, Jimenez JC, Wilson SF, et al. Complications after laparoscopic gastric bypass: a review of 3464 cases. Arch Surg 2003;138:957–61.
4. Bakhos C, Alkhoury F, Kyriakides T, et al. Early postoperative hemorrhage after open and laparoscopic roux-en-y gastric bypass. Obes Surg 2009;19:153–7.
5. Jamil LH, Krause KR, Chengelis DL, et al. Endoscopic management of early upper gastrointestinal hemorrhage following laparoscopic Roux-en-Y gastric bypass. Am J Gastroenterol 2008;103:86–91.
6. Bellorin O, Abdemur A, Sucandy I, et al. Understanding the significance, reasons and patterns of abnormal vital signs after gastric bypass for morbid obesity. Obes Surg 2010. [Epub ahead of print].
7. Papakonstantinou A, Terzis L, Stratopoulos C, et al. Bleeding from the upper gastrointestinal tract after Mason's vertical banded gastroplasty. Obes Surg 2000;10:582–4.

8. Pérez EM, Larrañaga E, Serrano P. Bleeding gastric pouch ulcer after vertical banded gastroplasty: a rare complication. Obes Surg 1997;7:454.
9. Iqbal M, Manjunath S, Seenath M, et al. Massive upper gastrointestinal hemorrhage: an unusual presentation after laparoscopic adjustable gastric banding due to erosion into the celiac axis. Obes Surg 2008;18:759–60.
10. Iannelli A, Dainese R, Piche T, et al. Laparoscopic sleeve gastrectomy for morbid obesity. World J Gastroenterol 2008;14:821–7.
11. Morino M, Toppino M, Forestieri P, et al. Mortality after bariatric surgery: analysis of 13,871 morbidly obese patients from a national registry. Ann Surg 2007;246: 1002–7.
12. Stein PD, Beemath A, Olson RE. Obesity as a risk factor in venous thromboembolism. Am J Med 2005;118:978–80.
13. Abdollahi M, Cushman M, Rosendaal FR. Obesity: risk of venous thrombosis and the interaction with coagulation factor levels and oral contraceptive use. Thromb Haemost 2003;89:493–8.
14. Goldhaber SZ, Tapson VF. A prospective registry of 5,451 patients with ultrasound-confirmed deep vein thrombosis. Am J Cardiol 2004;93:259–62.
15. Geerts WH, Pineo GF, Heit JA, et al. Prevention of venous thromboembolism: the seventh ACCP conference on antithrombotic and thrombolytic therapy. Chest 2004;126:338S–400S.
16. Pieracci FM, Barie PS, Pomp A. Critical care of the bariatric patient. Crit Care Med 2006;34:1796–804.
17. Nguyen NT, Goldman C, Rosenquist CJ, et al. Laparoscopic versus open gastric bypass: a randomized study of outcomes, quality of life, and costs. Ann Surg 2001;234:279–89.
18. Angrisani L, Furbetta F, Doldi SB, et al. Lap band adjustable gastric banding system: the Italian experience with 1863 patients operated on 6 years. Surg Endosc 2003;17:409–12.
19. Le Roux CW, Aylwin SJ, Batterham RL, et al. Gut hormone profiles following bariatric surgery favor an anorectic state, facilitate weight loss, and improve metabolic parameters. Ann Surg 2006;243:108–14.
20. Kothari SN, Lambert PJ, Mathiason MA. A comparison of thromboembolic and bleeding events following laparoscopic gastric bypass in patients treated with prophylactic regimens of unfractionated heparin or enoxaparin. Am J Surg 2007;194:709–11.
21. Caruana JA, McCabe MN, Smith AD, et al. Risk of massive upper gastrointestinal bleeding in gastric bypass patients taking clopidogrel. Surg Obes Relat Dis 2007;3:443–5.
22. Paige JT, Gouda BP, Gaitor-Stampley V, et al. No correlation between anti-factor Xa levels, low-molecular-weight heparin, and bleeding after gastric bypass. Surg Obes Relat Dis 2007;3:469–75.
23. Magee CJ, Barry J, Javed S, et al. Extended thromboprophylaxis reduces incidence of postoperative venous thromboembolism in laparoscopic bariatric surgery. Surg Obes Relat Dis 2010;6:322–5.
24. Greer IA, Gibson JL, Young A, et al. Effect of ketorolac and low-molecular-weight heparin individually and in combination on haemostasis. Blood Coagul Fibrinolysis 1999;10:367–73.
25. Petrusewicz J, Turowski M, Foks H, et al. Comparative studies of antiplatelet activity of nonsteroidal antiinflammatory drugs and new pyrazine CH- and NH-acids. Life Sci 1995;56:667–77.

26. Spaw AT, Husted JD. Bleeding after laparoscopic gastric bypass: case report and literature review. Surg Obes Relat Dis 2005;1:99–103.
27. Kaplan LM. Gastrointestinal management of the bariatric surgery patient. Gastroenterol Clin North Am 2005;34:105–25.
28. Rosenthal RJ, Szomstein S, Kennedy CI, et al. Laparoscopic surgery for morbid obesity: 1,001 consecutive bariatric operations performed at the Bariatric Institute, Cleveland Clinic Florida. Obes Surg 2006;16:119–24.
29. Chousleb E, Szomstein S, Podkameni D, et al. Routine abdominal drains after laparoscopic Roux-en-Y gastric bypass: a restrospective review of 593 patients. Obes Surg 2004;14:1203–7.
30. Nguyen NT, Rivers R, Wolfe BM. Early gastrointestinal hemorrhage after laparoscopic gastric bypass. Obes Surg 2003;13:62–5.
31. Huang CS, Farraye FA. Endoscopy in the bariatric surgical patient. Gastroenterol Clin North Am 2005;34:151–66.
32. Madan AK, Kuykendall SJ 4th, Ternovits CA, et al. Mallory-Weiss tear after laparoscopic Roux-en-Y gastric bypass. Surg Obes Relat Dis 2005;1:500–2.
33. Moreels TG, Hubens GJ, Ysebaert DK, et al. Diagnostic and therapeutic double-balloon enteroscopy after small bowel Roux-en-Y reconstructive surgery. Digestion 2009;80:141–7.
34. Tang SJ, Rivas H, Tang L, et al. Endoscopic hemostasis using endoclip in early gastrointestinal hemorrhage after gastric bypass surgery. Obes Surg 2007;17:1261–7.
35. Suggs WJ, Kouli W, Lupovici M, et al. Complications at gastrojejunostomy after laparoscopic Roux-en-Y gastric bypass: comparison between 21- and 25-mm circular staplers. Surg Obes Relat Dis 2007;3:508–14.
36. Moretto M, Mottin CC, Padoin AV, et al. Endoscopic management of bleeding after gastric bypas—a therapeutic alternative. Obes Surg 2004;14:706.
37. Steffen R. Early gastrointestinal hemorrhage after laparoscopic gastric bypass. Obes Surg 2003;13:466–7.
38. Jensen DM, Machicado GA, Hirabayashi K. Randomized controlled study of 3 different types of hemoclips for hemostasis of bleeding canine acute gastric ulcers. Gastrointest Endosc 2006;64:768–73.

Management of Postsurgical Leaks in the Bariatric Patient

Mario P. Morales, MD[a,*], Brent W. Miedema, MD[b], J. Stephen Scott, MD[a], Roger A. de la Torre, MD[b]

KEYWORDS

• Gastric bypass • Leak • Sepsis • Bariatrics • Complications • Stents • Endoscopy

Surgery is the most effective modality to treat morbid obesity, as reported by Pories and colleagues,[1] who rigorously followed more than 600 patients over a period of 16 years, demonstrating that gastric bypass produced durable weight loss greater than 100 lb and successful control of comorbidities. The application of laparoscopic techniques first described by Wittgrove and Clark[2] has led to a dramatic increase in the demand and use of surgery to treat morbid obesity. The number of annual bariatric procedures has steadily increased, reaching more than 100,000 in 2003.[3] This increase in the use of bariatric surgery carries with it an expected increase in the absolute number of surgical complications. Among the most devastating complications is that of a postsurgical leak. Diagnosis of these leaks can be difficult because of the lack of clinic signs and symptoms in this population. Morbidly obese patients also have comorbid conditions that further contribute to postoperative morbidity.

Pulmonary embolism is responsible for the majority of postoperative bariatric deaths.[4] If not fatal, pulmonary emboli are treated with anticoagulation and do not greatly increase hospital morbidity. In contrast, bariatric leaks often result in a systemic illness that prolongs hospital stay and may lead to multisystem organ failure that can be fatal. Postsurgical leaks produce a 2-fold increase in mortality and a 6-times increase in hospital stay compared with patients without leaks.[5]

Dr Miedema has received research funding from Boston Scientific and Alveolus (purchased by Merit Medical Systems). The other authors have nothing to disclose.

[a] SSM Weight-Loss Institute, DePaul Health Center, SSM Health Care, 12266 DePaul Drive Suite 310, St Louis, MO 63044, USA

[b] Department of General Surgery, University Hospital, University of Missouri, Columbia, MO 65212, USA

* Corresponding author. SSM Weight-Loss Institute, DePaul Health Center, SSM Health Care, 12266 DePaul Drive Suite 310, St Louis, MO 63044.

E-mail address: mpmoralesmd@yahoo.com

Gastrointest Endoscopy Clin N Am 21 (2011) 295–304

doi:10.1016/j.giec.2011.02.008 giendo.theclinics.com

1052-5157/11/$ – see front matter

The development of covered esophageal stents has provided a new tool in the treatment of postsurgical leaks. These removable stents can decrease hospital stay and simplify management of this patient group. The aim of this article is to discuss the current diagnosis and treatment of postsurgical leaks in bariatric patients.

CAUSES

Postsurgical leaks in bariatric patients generally occur at locations where a transection or anastomosis is made. These include the gastrojejunal anastomosis, the gastric pouch staple line, the gastric remnant staple line, the jejunojejunostomy, and, in the case of the duodenal switch, the duodeno-ileal staple line. The cause of bariatric leaks is unclear but likely secondary to technical factors, including anastomotic tension, tissue ischemia, and staple line sizing as well as anatomic variations of tissue thickness and blood supply. Various techniques have been described to limit tension on the gastrojejunal anastomosis. Scott and de la Torre[6] described positioning the Roux limb in the vertically divided omentum as a method with which to alleviate tension on the Roux limb at the gastrojejunal anastomosis. Higa and colleagues[7] describe retrocolic techniques that minimize the distance the Roux limb must extend in attaching to the gastric pouch. Fernandez and colleagues[8] reported that older age, male gender, and sleep apnea were all statistically significant independent variables in groups experiencing a postsurgical leak versus those that did not.

INCIDENCE

Leaks after bariatric surgery occur in approximately 1% to 6% of patients. A recent review reports 2.05% to 5.2% for laparoscopic Roux-en-Y gastric bypass (RYGB) and 1.68% to 2.6% for open RYGB. Additionally, sleeve gastrectomy has an associated leak rate up to 5.1%.[8–12] The frequency with which leaks occur at different sites is not specified in most studies. A study by Ballesta and colleagues[10] reported their experience regarding bariatric leaks by specific location: 68% at the gastrojejunostomy, 10% at the gastric pouch staple line, 3% at the remnant stomach staple line, 5% at the jejunojejunostomy, and the remaining 14% at combinations of these. Carruci and colleagues[11] reported that in 48 patients from 906 primary RYGB operations, 77% of leaks occurred at the gastrojejunal anastomosis, whereas the remaining leaks were at the blind limb, jejunjejunostomy, and remnant gastric staple line. In general, it is accepted that the gastrojejunostomy anastomosis is the site most prone to leak, because it is the most commonly noted site in many large series.[4,9]

DIAGNOSIS

Bariatric leaks are feared in part due to the challenge in making the diagnosis as well as the significant mortality rate that accompanies this complication. In some series, the death rate in patients presenting with a leak after bariatric procedures can be as high as 6%.[11] In contrast to the nonobese population, bariatric patients with a leak often present without fever, leukocytosis, or abdominal pain. These classic signs of viscous perforation are not reliable in the obese population. In addition, because of patient size, available radiographic imaging options, including upper gastrointestinal imaging (UGI) and CT scans, are of limited quality. In many patients, the only sign of a postsurgical leak is sustained tachycardia. Gonzalez and colleagues[13] reported that tachycardia (>100) was the only consistently present indicator in 72% of patients with a confirmed leak. In this study, fever and leukocytosis were present in 62% and

48%, respectively. Carruci and colleagues[11] also noted that tachycardia was present in an overwhelming number (92%) of leak patients. Nausea and vomiting were the next most common symptoms in 81% of that study group.

The primary radiologic techniques used in the diagnosis of bariatric leaks are UGI and CT scans. Because of patient obesity, both of these tests have limited diagnostic sensitivity[13,14] when used on routine basis; nevertheless, these studies do have a high predictive value when they are positive. Despite these limitations, radiologic evaluation is important in the early detection of leaks in the postoperative setting.[15] The primary diagnostic tool used to assess for postoperative leaks is a UGI study with an oral water-soluble contrast. This study is typically performed on postoperative day 1 or 2 and has shown variable sensitivity in detecting leaks. Reports as low as 33% leak detection have been published when UGI study is used routinely after gastric bypass operation.[14] This is likely because many leaks occur after a UGI study has been performed. The greatest value of a UGI study is when it is done in patients with clinical suspicion for a leak. The sensitivity can be as high as 92% under these circumstances.[16] The administration of oral methylene blue dye and observation of drain output can also be useful if a drain is left intraoperatively. Because of these diagnostic dilemmas, bariatric surgeons must rely on a combination of clinical suspicion and radiographic and laboratory evidence as well as vital sign trends to determine the possibility of a leak.

Another diagnostic approach to bariatric leaks is prophylactic placement of a drain at the time of surgery. In one study, 24% of leaks were detected by the observation of possible enteral content in the drain fluid.[17] There remains much controversy on the use of drains and the duration of placement.

STANDARD TREATMENT

Management of bariatric leaks has traditionally consisted of drainage, antibiotics, and specialized nutrition. Choice of drainage procedures is typically dictated by the condition of a patient and the characteristic of the leak—contained or free. In patients with hemodynamic instability, a surgical approach is preferred. In some series, the reoperative approach has been reported to be as high as 80%.[11] This allows for abdominal washout, possible attempts at repair or patch, and placement of appropriate drains. It also provides the opportunity to obtain enteral access for nutrition. The disadvantages of this approach include wound infection, dehiscence, hernia, feeding tube complications, and abdominal compartment syndrome. In a hemodynamically stable patient with controlled sepsis, a percutaneous approach is preferred if radiographically accessible. This avoids the morbidity associated with an additional operation although it negates the opportunity for feeding tube placement. Nutritional alternatives in these patients are typically limited to the total parenteral route. Parenteral nutrition is not optimal due to its expense and inherent risks of vascular thrombosis and line sepsis and lower efficacy compared with enteral feedings.

In recent years there has been an increase in the nonoperative management of leaks after gastric bypass as most leaks are well contained and do not require operative control. In one series of 46 bariatric leaks, 40 were contained.[17] Of these contained leaks, 33 could be treated without reoperation. Nonoperative treatment consisted of nothing by mouth, antibiotics, and specialized nutrition. Serial UGI studies were performed until radiologic closure was documented. Using this approach, radiologic resolution of the leak occurred at a median of 17 days, when oral intake could be started. There was no mortality in this study. The nonoperative strategy in this study required the drain to be left in place at least 1 week after surgery.

THE USE OF STENTS

A possible adjunct in managing postsurgical leaks involves minimally invasive techniques using stents placed with endoscopic and fluoroscopic guidance. Covered stents can be placed in the bowel lumen at the site of the leak in a minimally invasive fashion. Stents offer several treatment advantages that can simplify surgical management of postoperative leaks. A stent prevents or greatly diminishes further peritoneal contamination by excluding the leak site from enteral secretions. This in turn is thought to promote and accelerate leak healing. Stent placement results in a rapid improvement in abdominal pain as a result of decreased peritoneal contamination. Shielding of the leak site also permits nutrition to be given orally in many cases. Parenteral nutrion is seldom necessary. **Fig. 1** illustrates prestent and poststent treatment of a gastroejunal anastomotic leak.

Early stents were rigid and primarily used to bypass malignant narrowing of the esophagus or colon. These stents generally required operative placement and were associated with a high morbidity. A significant improvement was the development of meshed expandable metal stents that could be placed under endoscopic and/or fluoroscopic control. Tumors would sometimes grow through the gaps in meshed stents and again obstruct the bowel lumen. Thus, a silicone covering of the stent was introduced to prevent tissue ingrowth and reobstruction from tumors. It was soon discovered that these types of covered stents could be retrieved at a later date and thus could be used as temporary stents for nonmalignant conditions.[18,19] These temporary removable stents were subsequently used successfully in the treatment of anastamotic complications of the esophagus. Only recently (2006) have there been reports of using covered stents temporarily for complications of bariatric surgery (ie, postsurgical leaks).[20–22]

Current covered stents have an inner mesh cannula made of nitinol or polyester. These stents are designed to be compressed and are packaged in a removable sheath as part of the delivery system. When the sheath is withdrawn, the stent expands to a predetermined size and with a radial force that is designed to avoid bowel perforation. At luminal sites of bowel stenosis, the stent often does not fully expand due to counter force from the fibrotic rigidity at the stricture site. An outer coat of silicone

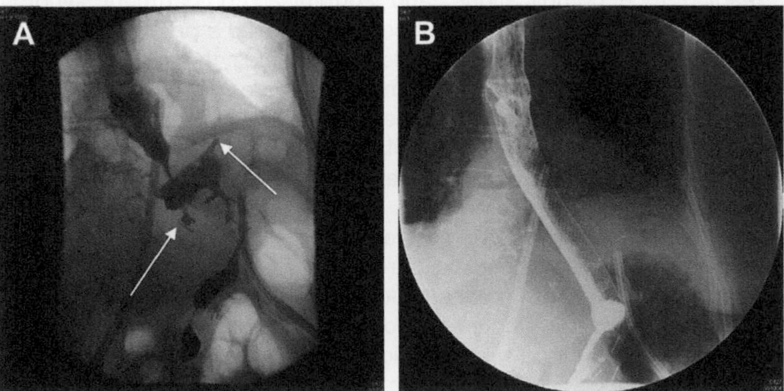

Fig. 1. (*A*) Anastamotic leak at the gastrojejunostomy after RYGB. Arrows show the site of leaking contrast. (*B*) UGI study after stent placement in the same patient.

is impermeable and prevents intestinal mucosa and fibrotic tissues from being incorporated into the gaps in the stent. This property allows the stents to be removed, usually within 8 weeks.

Several innovations have been developed in an attempt to decrease the rate of stent migration. Most covered stents include a proximal flare with an increase in diameter of 3 to 5 mm over a length of approximately 2 cm. Some stents also include a distal flare. The Alimaxx (Merit Medical Systems, Merit Endotek, South Jordan, UT, USA) stent has short barbs on the external surface. These barbs are oriented distally so as to impale the mucosa in a tangential fashion and thus help hold the stent in place. Boston Scientific (Boston Scientific Endoscopy, Marlborough, MA, USA) also has partially covered stents where the proximal 3 cm of the stent is left bare. This results in mucosal ingrowth through the gaps of the bare portion of the stent. In a few days, the stents are firmly held in place by tissue ingrowth. Removal may later be achieved in some cases by stent inversion. Alternatively, removal may require placement of a second fully covered stent within the initial partially covered stent, to provide pressure necrosis of the ingrown tissue, with subsequent simultaneous removal of both stents a few days later. Other investigators have advocated the use of fibrin glue and stents together to help improve successful closure.[20]

The authors' experience with stents dates back to January of 2007. The authors have reported the largest experience describing stents for treatment of bariatric surgery complications, involving 26 patients treated with 55 endoscopic stent procedures.[23] In this report, patients with gastrointestinal (GI) leaks were treated with endoscopically placed polyester (Polyflex, Boston Scientific) or nitinol (Alimaxx-E, Merit Endotek) stents. Both of these stents were completely covered with a silicone coating.

In this experience, the authors used stent treatment in 17 patients with GI leaks. On average, each patient received stent treatment three separate times. Seven patients only received one stent. The mean operative time for stent evaluation and placement was 63 minutes.

Rapid symptom improvement was seen in 94% of patients, and 92% received oral nutrition within 24 hours of stent placement. The mean time from first stent placement to final stent removal was 40 days. Leak resolution occurred in 16 of 17 patients and was durable out to a mean of 15 months. Two patients developed strictures that responded to placement of another stent. In the one failure, the leak did not resolve with stenting and revisional surgery was required for final resolution. This one failure occurred early in the series and was likely due to poor control of peritoneal contamination.

STENT PLACEMENT TECHNIQUE

The authors' technique for stent placement has become standardized. Both endoscopy and fluoroscopy techniques are used to place stents. The authors feel this gives better control and more precise positioning of the stent. The procedure is done with patients under general tracheal anesthesia in a supine position. Broad-spectrum antibiotics are given if a patient has not yet received them. A standard upper endoscope (GIF-H160, Olympus, Center Valley, PA, USA) is used.

The endoscope is initially passed to the site of the leak. The leak can be seen endoscopically approximately 50% of the time. The endoscope is then introduced at least 40 cm down the Roux limb or to the third portion of the duodenum for sleeve gastrectomy patients. A floppy guide wire is then passed through the biopsy channel of the endoscope. The scope is then withdrawn to the site of the leak. Fluoroscopy is then used to mark the site of the leak and the squamocolumnar junction with an external metal marker (**Fig. 2**B). The scope is then removed leaving the guide wire in position.

A delivery system with a stent of 22 to 23 mm in diameter and 12 to 15 cm in length is then placed over the wire and into position under fluoroscopic control (see **Fig. 2**C). Occasionally the delivery system cannot be negotiated around an acute angle. This can usually be resolved by switching to a stiff (Savary-Gilliard, Cook Medical, Winston-Salem, NC, USA) guide wire.

The stent is then deployed under continuous fluoroscopy. The stent is released from distal to proximal. The release of the distal portion of the stent is initiated at least 5 cm distal to the leak (see **Fig. 2**D). The delivery system is removed and the stent is viewed

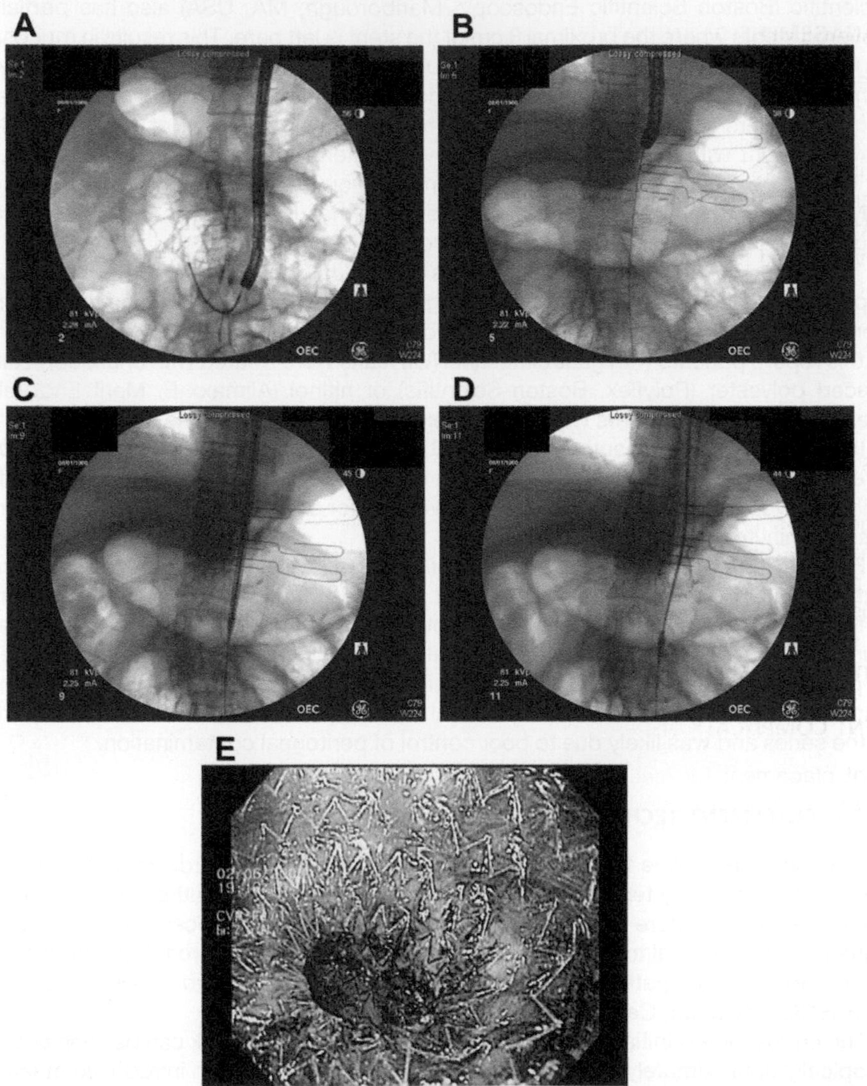

Fig. 2. (*A*) Placement of the guide wire deep in the Roux limb under fluoroscopic guidance. (*B*) Radioopaque markers to identify the location of the leak and the squamocolumnar junction between the esophagus and the stomach. (*C*) Positioning the stent delivery sytem under fluoroscopy. (*D*) Position of stent after deployment. Arrows show the position of the stent. (*E*) Endoscopic verification of stent placement.

endoscopically (see **Fig. 2**E). If the stent is not in the correct position, adjustment is done using a flexible short tip rat tooth forceps placed through the biopsy channel of the endoscope. The proximal suture or one of the distal loops on the stent is grasped and the stent repositioned. It is often necessary to treat distal strictures, if present, to achieve a successful leak treatment.

The goal proximally is to have at least 5 cm of the distal esophagus stented. This may require placement of a second stent with a 5-cm to 8-cm overlap with the first stent. Finally, endoscopic evaluation and measurements are done. Rarely, a third stent is used to make sure an adequate length of the esophagus is stented.

MANAGEMENT OF THE STENT PATIENT

After stent placement, patients are kept on nothing by mouth status until the next morning. A GI study using 15 mL of a water contrast solution is repeated 3 times. If the leak is sealed, patients are started on liquids and the bariatric diet is advanced, as in patients without a leak. When the leak is sealed, patients are generally discharged the day after the diet is started.

After discharge, patients have a weekly abdominal radiograph to monitor for stent movement. If stent migration is seen, patients undergo endoscopy and the stent is repositioned or removed. The goal is to leave the stent in place 4 weeks to allow adequate time for leak closure. This stent is sometimes removed sooner due to intolerance. Early stent removal is followed by a UGI water contrast study. Resumption of diet is based on the result of this study. If a stent has been in more than 3 weeks, a liquid diet is started immediately after stent removal. Radiographic healing is documented a mean of 6 days after stent removal.

Stent removal is also done under general endotracheal anesthesia to minimize the risk of aspiration. The stents have a circumferential suture placed at the proximal edge. This suture is grasped and pulled proximal causing the proximal end of the stent to narrow. The stent is then slowly removed with constant pressure. Additional stents are removed in a similar manner. Suture breakage was common with early stents but is unusual with the current generation of stents. If the suture breaks, a proximal loop of the stent is grasped and slowly removed under direct vision. Alternating sides of the stent may need to be grasped for safe removal.

STENT COMPLICATIONS

Stent placement for leaks is currently associated with a high complication rate. It is common for patients to experience substernal chest pain with radiation to the back, and patients often have nausea that can be difficult to treat. Treatment with pain medication and multiple antiemetics for the most part controls patients' symptoms. Occasionally, however, the stent must be removed due to intolerable symptoms.

The most common complication is stent migration. In the authors' series of 55 endoscopic stent procedures, migration was seen in 22 (40%).[23] Most of these[18] could be recovered or repositioned by upper endoscopy. **Fig. 3** depicts a patient who initially had two overlapping stents. CT scan 2 weeks later demonstrates proximal and distal migration of the two stents. Two stents passed through the entire GI tract, however. The other 2 became lodged in the small bowel and required laparoscopic removal.

The authors were able to decrease the migration rate from 64% in the first 25 patients to 20% in the last 30. This was accomplished by using longer and overlapping stents. In addition, nitinol stents had a lower migration rate than polyester stents (48% vs 32%) and were used more frequently later in the study.

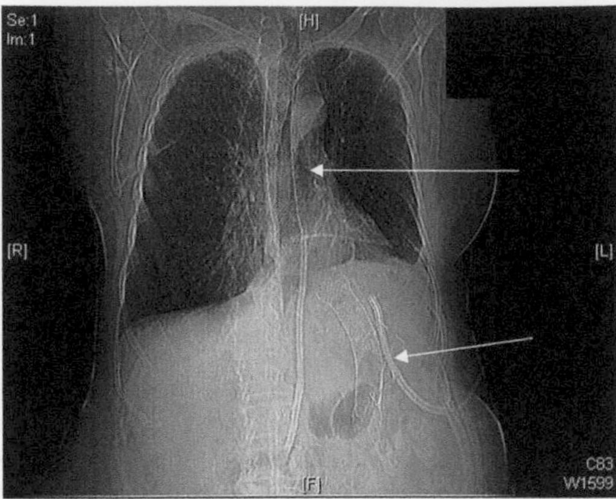

Fig. 3. Migration after stent placement. Arrows show proximal and distal stents completely separated after distal stent migration into small bowel.

The authors experienced four major complications. Early in the experience, a stent fractured and required tedious piecemeal extraction. One stent obstructed due to kinking and required replacement. The distal end of another stent created an enterotomy in the Roux limb that required laparoscopic repair. Finally, one stent could not be removed endoscopically due to mucosal incorporation and laparoscopic removal was needed.

More recently, the authors have been using a partially covered nitinol stent, the WallFlex partially covered esophageal stent (Boston Scientific). The proximal flare on the stent is uncovered for 3 cm, allowing mucosal and fibrotic incorporation into this portion of the stent. This mucosal tissue ingrowth results in anchoring the stent. In the authors' experience the metal partially covered stents resulted in less migration compared with covered stents. These stents can be difficult to remove, however, and can remove a 3-cm circumference of the bowel wall (**Fig. 4**).

FUTURE TREATMENTS

The authors believe that immediate stenting of a leak after bariatric surgery is superior to prior treatment approaches. Most stent technical problems (fracture, suture

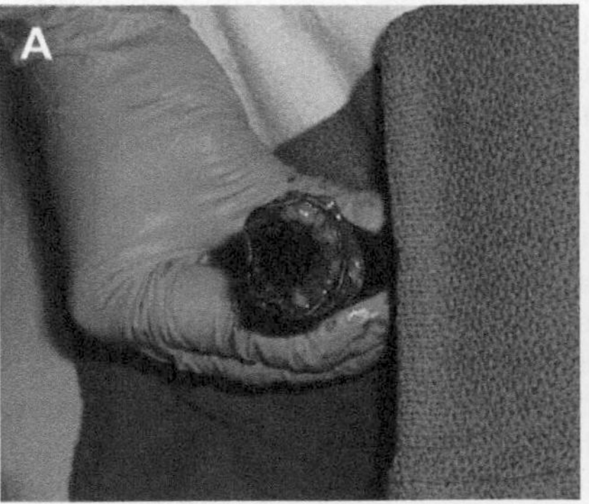

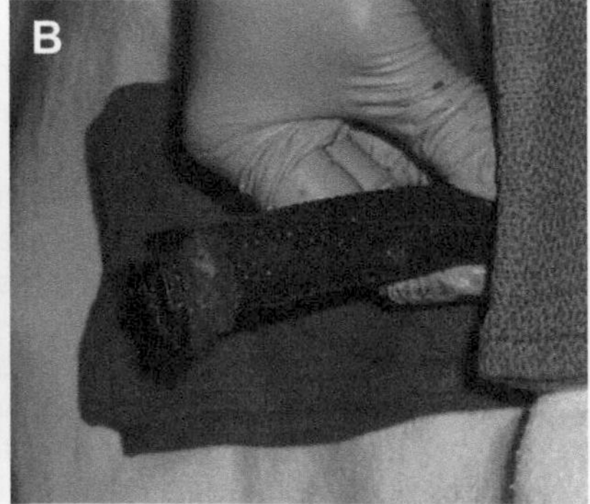

Fig. 4. (*A*) Circumferential tissue ingrowth that remains on the end of the proximal portion of a partially covered stent after removal. (*B*) Lateral view.

breakage, and tissue ingrowth) have been solved. The problem with migration continues, however. The authors have attempted to secure stents with endoscopic clips, bioabsorbable sutures to the bowel wall, and sutures attached to a stent and bridled at the nose. None of these has been satisfactory. Blackmon and colleagues[19] describe a suture pexy technique for stents that are positioned high in the esophagus. A suture needle passer instrument is introduced under ultrasound guidance through the lower lateral neck and into the stent lumen where a suture is endoscopically introduced. It would be much more difficult and risky, however, to use this technique for stents lower in the esophagus. A technical innovation is needed to solve this problem.

Another important advance would be to develop a stent with a bioabsorbable core. Once a stent begins to disintegrate, it could be passed harmlessly through the GI tract. This would obviate the risk and expense of stent retrieval.

The stent delivery systems have been getting progressively small in diameter. There is currently not a stent delivery system that can fit through the biopsy channel of an upper endoscope, however. If this could be accomplished, stents could be placed more precisely and using only endoscopy. This would also make multiple passes of the scope and delivery system unnecessary, allowing placement to be done safely under conscious sedation.

SUMMARY

Bariatric leaks occur in approximately 1% to 6% of patients after bariatric surgery. Symptoms are subtle and often result in a delay of diagnosis. Standard treatment is drainage of the leak, nothing by mouth, and specialized nutrition until the leak is healed. Endoscopic stent treatment of leaks after bariatric surgery is safe and effective. Stents allow early oral nutrition, decreased use of parenteral nutrition, decreased ICU stay, and a decreased hospital stay. Improved stent technology is needed to overcome the main complication of stent migration.

REFERENCES

1. Pories WJ, Swanson MS, MacDonald KG, et al. Who would have thought it? An operation proves to be the most effective terhapy for adult-onset diabetes mellitus. Ann Surg 1995;222:339–50.
2. Wittgrove AC, Clark GW. Laparoscopic gastric bypass, Roux-en-Y, 500 patients: technique and results, with 3-60 month follow up. Obes Surg 2000;10:233–9.
3. Santry HP, Gillen DL, Lauderdale DS. Trends in bariatric surgical procedures. JAMA 2005;294(15):1909–17.
4. Podnos YD, Jimenez JC, Wilson SE, et al. Complications after laparoscopic gastric bypass: a review of 3464 cases. Arch Surg 2003;138:957–61.
5. Almahmeed T, Gonzalez R, Nelson LG, et al. Morbidity of anastomotic leaks in patients undergoing Roux-en-Y gastric bypass. Arch Surg 2007;142(10):954–7.
6. Scott JS, de la Torre RA. Laparoscopic Roux-en-Y gastric bypass: a totally intra-abdominal approach—technique and preliminary report. Obes Surg 1999;9(5):492–8.
7. Higa KD, Boone KB, Ho T, et al. Laparoscopic Roux-en-Y gastric bypass for morbid obesity: technique and preliminary results of our first 400 patients. Arch Surg 2000;135(9):1029–33.
8. Fernandez AZ Jr, DeMaria EJ, Tichansky DS, et al. Experience with over 3,000 open and laparoscopic bariatric procedures: multivariate analysis of factors related to leak and resultant mortality. Surg Endosc 2004;18(2):193–7.

9. Higa KD, Boone KB, Ho T. Complications of the laparoscopic Roux-en-Y Gastric bypass: 1,040 patients—what have we learned? Obes Surg 2000;10:509–13.
10. Ballesta C, Berindoague R, Cabrera M, et al. Management of anastomotic leaks after laparoscopic Roux-en-Y gastric bypass. Obes Surg 2008;18(6):623–30.
11. Carucci LR, Turner MA, Conklin RC, et al. Roux-en-Y gastric bypass surgery for morbid obesity: evaluation of postoperative extraluminal leaks with upper gastrointestinal series. Radiology 2006;238(1):119–27.
12. Shaikh SN, Thompson CC. Treatment of leaks and fistula after bariatric surgery. Tech Gastrointest Endosc 2010;12(3):141–5.
13. Gonzalez R, Sarr MG, Smith CD, et al. Diagnosis and contemporary management of anastomotic leaks after gastric bypass for obesity. J Am Coll Surg 2007;204(1): 47–55.
14. Doraiswamy A, Rasmussen JJ, Pierce J, et al. The utility of routine postoperative upper GI series following laparoscopic gastric bypass. Surg Endosc 2007; 21(12):2159–62.
15. Ganci-Cerrud G, Herrera MF. Role of radiologic contrast studies in the early postoperative period after bariatric surgery. Obes Surg 1999;9(6):532–4.
16. Madan AK, Stoecklein HH, Ternovits CA, et al. Predictive value of upper gastrointestinal studies versus clinical signs for gastrointestinal leaks after laparoscopic gastric bypass. Surg Endosc 2007;21(2):194–6.
17. Thodiyil PA, Yenumula P, Rogula T, et al. Selective nonoperative management of leaks after gastric bypass: lessons learned from 2675 consecutive patients. Ann Surg 2008;248:782–92.
18. Eloubeidi MA, Lopes TL. Novel removable internally fully covered self-expaning metal esophageal stent: feasibility, technique of removal and tissue response in humans. Am J Gastroenterol 2009;104(6):1374–81.
19. Blackmon SH, Santora R. Utility of removable esophageal covered self-expanding metal stents for leak and fistula management. Ann Thorac Surg 2010;89:931–7.
20. Merrifield BF, Lautz D, Thompson CC. Endoscopic repair of gastric leaks after Roux-en-Y gastric bypass: a less invasive approach. Gastrointest Endosc 2006;63(4):710–4.
21. Eisendrath P, Cremer M, Himpens J, et al. Endotherapy including temporary stenting of fistulas of the upper gastrointestinal tract after laparoscopic bariatric surgery. Endoscopy 2007;39(7):625–30.
22. Thaler K. Treatment of leaks and other bariatric complications with endoluminal stents [review]. J Gastrointest Surg 2009;13(9):1567–9.
23. Iqbal A, Miedema BW, Ramaswamy A, et al. Long-term outcome after endoscopic stent therapy for complications after bariatric surgery. Surg Endosc 2011;25:505–20.

Accessing the Pancreatobiliary Limb and ERCP in the Bariatric Patient

Mouen A. Khashab, MD[a], Patrick I. Okolo III, MD, MPH[b,*]

KEYWORDS

- Roux-en-Y gastric bypass (RYGB)
- Double-balloon enteroscopy (DBE)
- Single-balloon enteroscopy (SBE) • Spiral enteroscopy (SE)
- Endoscopic retrograde cholangiopancreatography (ERCP)

The obesity epidemic and the high prevalence of obesity-related comorbidities have received considerable attention, and are currently considered a worldwide public health priority.[1–3] Behavioral and pharmacologic treatments have had limited efficacy, particularly in the setting of severe obesity. Surgical treatment of obesity has been established to be the only effective means of significant and sustainable weight loss in this patient population. Equally important, bariatric surgery can significantly improve obesity-related comorbidities and quality of life. Within the past decade, the volume of bariatric surgery has increased by 900% in the United States and 350% in other parts of the world.[4–7]

The Roux-en-Y gastric bypass (RYGB) accounts for more than 60% of bariatric procedures performed in the United States today.[6] The first step during RYGB surgeries is creation of a small gastric pouch approximately 30 mL in size. The jejunum is then divided into upper (biliopancreatic) and lower limbs, typically 30 to 60 cm distal to the ligament of Treitz, although some surgeons create much longer biliopancreatic limbs (100–150 cm). The Roux limb is brought up to the level of the gastric pouch and anastomosed to the gastric pouch (gastrojejunostomy). The biliopancreatic limb and

---

Conflicts of interest: M.A.K. has nothing to disclose; P.I.O. has disclosed a consultant relationship with Spirus Medical and Boston Scientific.

[a] Division of Gastroenterology and Hepatology, Department of Medicine, The Johns Hopkins Medical Institutions, Johns Hopkins University, 1830 East Monument Street, Room 1700A, Baltimore, MD 21205, USA

[b] Division of Gastroenterology and Hepatology, Department of Medicine, The Johns Hopkins Medical Institutions, Johns Hopkins University, 615 North Wolfe Street, Blalock Building, Suite 404, Baltimore, MD 21205, USA

* Corresponding author.

E-mail address: pokolo2@jhmi.edu

Gastrointest Endoscopy Clin N Am 21 (2011) 305–313
doi:10.1016/j.giec.2011.02.003 giendo.theclinics.com
1052-5157/11/$ – see front matter

Roux limb are connected via a jejunojejunostomy 75 to 150 cm distal to the gastrojejunostomy.[8] In fact, the longest Roux limbs are encountered in those created as part of RYGB procedures.

The performance of endoscopic retrograde cholangiopancreatography (ERCP) in the setting of RYGB is challenging. The first major challenge is the length of the bowel that has to be traversed to access the papilla. This frequently necessitates the use of forward-viewing enteroscopes to reach the papilla. The use of forward-viewing scopes to access the papilla and perform ERCP in these patients represents a challenge itself. The papillary orifice is not routinely visible using forward-viewing instruments. When the orifice is visible, its alignment with the scope and instruments used during ERCP is often suboptimal, especially in view of the absence of an elevator. Another hindrance is the sharp angulation at the jejunojejunostomy, which often requires an almost 180-degree U-turn to access the pancreaticobiliary limb. Finally, the performance of ERCP using enteroscopes requires the use of many specialized accessories, the availability of which may be limited in some markets.

INDICATIONS

Indications for ERCP in patients who are post-RYGB surgery encompass all indications for the procedure as in patients with native gastrointestinal anatomy. Some diseases, however, occur more often in RYGB patients. Rapid weight loss creates a lithogenic state and is associated with an increased risk of cholelithiasis. This results from increased bile mucin content and bile calcium concentration in the gallbladder during periods of weight loss.[9] Although the gallbladder is often removed during open RYGB, this is not a routine practice during laparoscopic RYGB. Also, papillary stenosis can be seen in this population, and often requires ERCP with endoscopic biliary sphincterotomy.

METHODS OF ACCESSING THE PAPILLA IN RYGB PATIENTS

Multiple studies have assessed the use of different techniques to access the papilla in patients with altered anatomy. Although some of these studies investigated patients who have undergone Roux-en-Y reconstructive surgeries, none focused on bariatric RYGB patients. The RYGB surgical anatomy represents a particular challenge to endoscopists who intend to perform papillary interventions because it entails creation of the longest Roux limbs for purposes of weight loss.

ERCP Using Duodenoscopes and Colonoscopes

The side-viewing duodenoscope is the optimal instrument to perform ERCP because of the location of the ampulla on the medial side of the duodenum. Nevertheless, advancement of the duodenoscope through the anatomic route to reach the ampulla in RYGB patients is almost impossible. Hintze and colleagues[10] reported a failure rate of 67% to reach the ampulla using a duodenoscope in patients with Roux-en-Y anatomy (none post-RYGB). This failure rate is expected to be higher in RYGB patients who usually have longer Roux limbs. Wright and colleagues[11] used a pediatric colonoscope to access the afferent limb and place a guide wire, followed by advancement of the duodenoscope over the wire using fluoroscopic guidance. ERCP was possible in 45% of patients with RYGB anatomy. Therefore, the use of a duodenoscope to perform ERCP in RYGB patients frequently fails. In addition, this technique should be attempted only by experienced endoscopists because of the challenge of navigating a side-viewing instrument through altered anatomy, for a long distance, through anastomoses, and through sharp angulations.

ERCP Using Double-Balloon Enteroscopy

Three types of endoscopes (and overtubes) for double-balloon enteroscopy (DBE) (Fujinon, Inc, Saitama, Japan) are currently available. The EN-450P5 (effective length 2 m, outer diameter 8.5 mm, biopsy channel diameter 2.2 mm) is mainly used for diagnostic purposes. The EN-450T5 (effective length 2 m, outer diameter 9.4 mm, biopsy channel diameter 2.8 mm) can be used for diagnostic and therapeutic indications. The EC-450BI5 (effective length 1.52 m, outer diameter 9.4 mm, biopsy channel diameter 2.8 mm) has a shorter working length. This shorter scope is ideal to use for accessing the papilla in RYGB patients because all standard ERCP accessories, some of which are too short to use with a 2-m scope, can be used. The DBE enteroscope is advanced in the small bowel as previously described by Yamamoto and colleagues.[12,13]

Sakai and colleagues[14] were the first to use DBE for the evaluation of the bypassed stomach after RYGB. Since then, multiple studies have described the use of DBE to facilitate the performance of ERCP in patients with Roux-en-Y anatomy.[15–23] These studies reported a high success rate of greater than 90% for reaching the biliopancreatic limb and an 80% success rate for ERCP. However, most of the subjects studied were not bariatric RYGB patients. Emmett and Mallat[17] performed DBE-ERCP in patients with Roux-en-Y anatomy. The ampulla was reached in all patients after Roux-en-Y and ERCP was successful in 88% of these patients. Although these results are encouraging, most of the reported data and experience comes from studying patients with hepaticojejunostomy. These patients have shorter Roux limbs. In addition, cannulation of hepaticojejunostomy anastomosis is less technically demanding than cannulation of a native ampulla, especially when these are approached in retrograde fashion.

ERCP Using Single-Balloon Enteroscopy

Single-balloon enteroscopy (SBE) and spiral enteroscopy (SE) are the latest breakthrough techniques in endoscopic evaluation of the small bowel. SBE has been introduced to simplify the technique of push-and-pull enteroscopy.[24–26] Some investigators have suggested that SBE is more intuitive to learn and possibly more efficient than DBE.[24] The potential advantages of SBE over DBE include shorter setup time, 1 balloon cycle requirement instead of 2, a less cumbersome balloon control panel, a less floppy scope, and the use of a nonlatex balloon.[27] The single-balloon overtube (Olympus Optical, Tokyo, Japan) is used for SBE procedures. The overtube has one balloon at its tip and both the balloon and overtube are made of silicone. The overtube measures 140 cm in length and has a diameter of 13.2 mm. The enteroscope is advanced to its maximal position without looping and the overtube is then advanced to the distal portion of the enteroscope. The scope tip is either deflected into a U-turn to hook onto the SB mucosa or the mucosa is suctioned to stabilize the scope position. After inflating the balloon, the assembly is withdrawn. This series of maneuvers is then repeated until the anatomic area of interest is reached or when the endoscopist deems further maneuvers will not result in significant advancement of the scope.

Few studies, none of which was dedicated to study RYGB patients, have evaluated the use of SBE in patients with Roux-en-Y anatomy.[28–30] Itoi and colleagues[28] evaluated the usefulness of SBE-ERCP in 11 patients with Roux-en-Y anastomosis, none of which represented RYGB anatomy. The papilla was reached in 91% of these patients and ERCP was successfully performed in 73% of them. Dellon and colleagues[29] reported on 4 patients with Roux-en-Y anatomy who underwent SBE. One patient after RYGB underwent successful SBE-ERCP for abnormal liver enzymes and jaundice. Wang and colleagues[30] assessed the effectiveness of SBE-ERCP in 13 patients with altered anatomy, 6 of whom were post-RYGB. The ampulla was reached and ERCP was successful in 4 of these patients. The ampulla could not be reached on the first attempt in 2 patients because of a tight hairpin turn that was required to reach and intubate the afferent limb from the Roux-en-Y anastomosis. In both patients, a second SBE-ERCP was attempted and was successful.

ERCP Using Spirus Enteroscopy

Spirus enteroscopy (SE) is performed using the Endo-Ease Discovery SB overtube (Spirus Medical, Stoughton, MA, USA). The overtube is made of polyvinyl chloride and measures 118 cm with a 21-cm spiral element at the tip. Advancement is made by clockwise rotation until the point of depth of maximal insertion. The enteroscope is then unlocked from the overtube and advanced as far as possible. The enteroscope is subsequently withdrawn in a similar manner to the previously mentioned "hook-and-suction technique," while rotating the overtube. This sequence is repeated about 3 times. Withdrawal is performed by counterclockwise rotation of the overtube.

One study published only in abstract form described a single-center experience with SE in 57 patients, 7 of whom were post-RYGB. The excluded stomach was reached in 5 of these patients. No further details were provided.[31]

ERCP Through Gastrostomy or Jejunostomy Tracts

Baron and Vickers[32] were first to describe creation of a surgical gastrostomy to facilitate ERCP in an RYGB patient who had failed an attempt at ERCP using an enteroscope through the anatomic route. Since then, multiple other investigators have described their similar experience with high success rates.[33,34] The technique involves initial placement of a surgical gastrostomy in the excluded stomach. ERCP is then performed at a later time through a healed gastrostomy tract. The gastrostomy tube is removed, followed by passage of a forward-viewing scope through the tract. Wire-guided Savary dilation of the tract is then performed. The duodenoscope is passed through the dilated tract to the duodenum and ERCP is performed in the usual manner.

Although gastrostomy offers a reliable means to perform ERCP in RYGB patients, this technique is more invasive than the previously described endoscopic techniques, and entails surgical and anesthesia risks. In addition, gastrostomy tubes negatively affect the quality of life of patients and should be removed as soon as repeat ERCP is deemed unnecessary.[35] Another limitation of this technique is that it is sometimes impractical to wait for the gastrostomy tract to mature before performing ERCP (such as in patients with acute cholangitis or severe acute biliary pancreatitis).

Baron[36] described the technique of retrograde placement of percutaneous endoscopic gastrostomy (RPEG) to allow subsequent ERCP in patients with RYGB who have failed prior attempts at ERCP via the anatomic route. With this technique, the endoscope is advanced proximal to the ampulla and into the excluded stomach in retrograde fashion. An area of transillumination and indentation for RPEG is identified and the procedure is then completed in the usual fashion.

Laparoscopic-Assisted ERCP

Laparoscopic-assisted ERCP in RYGB patients refers to the laparoscopic creation of a point of access to the gastric remnant for the duodenoscope to reach the papilla. This technique may be used in patients with RYGB who had failed prior attempts at accessing the papilla using the previously described methods. Although laparoscopic-assisted ERCP is not widely practiced, several recent studies that assessed the use of this technique have reported encouraging results.[37–39]

Initial surgical access to the abdomen is gained by using a Veress needle. A shielded trocar is inserted, and a laparoscopic examination is then conducted. The ligament of Treitz is identified, which allows identification of the afferent Roux limb. The bowel is then followed distally from the Y connection. The biliopancreatic limb is occluded with a bowel clamp to prevent insufflation of the gastrointestinal tract, which obscures laparoscopic visualization. A 15-mm trocar is introduced into the left upper quadrant through which the sterilized duodenoscope is passed. The endoscopist guides the endoscope through the 15-mm trocar and monitors it as it exits into the peritoneum. The surgeon and endoscopist work together to guide the endoscope into the excluded stomach. Once into the excluded stomach, the endoscope is advanced through the pylorus and positioned in the second duodenum, and ERCP is performed in the usual fashion.

Lopes and colleagues[39] recently reported their experience with laparoscopic-assisted ERCP in 10 patients. Biliary cannulation was successful in 90% of cases. The investigators also recognized and treated 4 internal hernias during laparoscopic examination. All of the hernias were missed on preoperative CT examination. Tension pneumothorax developed in one patient during the procedure, which was caused by an indwelling percutaneous transhepatic cholangiography (PTC) catheter that crossed the diaphragm. This was promptly recognized and treated successfully with chest tube placement.

CHOOSING THE OPTIMAL TECHNIQUE

The technique of choice to perform ERCP in patients who are post-RYGB is best dictated by local expertise. Other factors, such as acuity, results of prior ERCP attempts, surgical risk, need for multiple ERCP procedures, length of Roux limb, possibility of internal hernias, and patient's preference may also play a role in choosing the optimal technique. Device-assisted enteroscopy techniques (DBE, SBE, and SE) are the least invasive and the most studied and established techniques for this purpose. However, their performance is technically demanding, time consuming, and often requires the availability of specialized accessories. Other techniques are best used in patients who fail deep enteroscopy-assisted ERCP. Patients who may require repeated elective ERCP procedures are best served by placement of a temporary gastrostomy. Laparoscopic-assisted ERCP may be used in patients who are suspected of having internal hernias at centers with experience in this technique.

DEEP ENTEROSCOPY-ASSISTED ERCP: ADVANCEMENT AND CANNULATION TECHNIQUES

The enteroscopy system device (enteroscope and overtube) is advanced to the jejunojejunostomy as described previously. The first challenge at the anastomosis is to identify the pancreaticobiliary limb. At the anastomosis, the endoscopist typically visualizes 2 or 3 lumens into which the endoscope may be passed. One of these lumens represents a blind end as a result of an end-to-side anastomosis. The second lumen leads into the efferent limb and the third leads into the afferent (pancreaticobiliary) limb. There is no reliable method to correctly identify the afferent limb and bile might be present in both. The passage identified directly adjacent to the blind end is usually the common limb. The biliopancreatic limb is usually situated at an almost 180-degree turn once the endoscope is inserted into the Roux-en-Y anastomosis. Consequently, intubation of this limb is challenging and may require the performance of a “U-turn.” If this maneuver is repeatedly unsuccessful, changing the patient's position and/or applying abdominal pressure may be of benefit. The use of fluoroscopy may help in identifying the biliopancreatic limb. When the common channel is intubated inadvertently, fluoroscopy will reveal formation of multiple intestinal loops in the pelvis. We frequently inject dye through an ERCP catheter to obtain an enterographic study of the small bowel. This helps delineate the anatomy and may aid in identifying whether the endoscope is in the biliopancreatic or the common limb. When the common limb is unintentionally intubated, the enteroscope should be withdrawn slowly to the level of the anastomosis. A tattoo or a clip may be placed in the common limb just past the anastomosis to prevent inadvertent reintubation of the common limb.

If intubation of the biliopancreatic limb fails because of a tight turn at the anastomosis, a long retrieval balloon catheter and a long guide wire can be deployed deeply into the biliopancreatic limb under fluoroscopic guidance. This maneuver stiffens the enteroscope and provides countertraction, which may enable successful advancement of the enteroscope into the biliopancreatic limb and subsequent access to the ampulla.[30]

Initially, when balloon-assisted enteroscopy is used, the enteroscope should be passed alone (without the overtube) across the anastomosis and advanced into the biliopancreatic limb as far as possible. The enteroscope is then affixed to the biliopancreatic limb by inflating the balloon on the enteroscope (for DBE) or by using the "turn and suction technique" (for SBE) before the overtube is pushed around the angled anastomosis. The enteroscope/overtube system should then be shortened as much as possible to free up a sufficient length of scope around the angle at the ligament of Treitz.

Cannulation of the major papilla, as mentioned previously, can represent a major challenge to the endoscopist for several reasons. The use of forward-viewing scopes to access the papilla may impede its complete visualization. In addition, this may create difficulties in terms of proper angle of approach for cannulation, especially in view of the absence of an elevator. Also, the retrograde access to the ampulla results in an inverted orientation of the papilla. Finally, some long ERCP accessories need to be custom ordered and are not widely available in all markets. These include needle knives, sphincterotomes, retrieval balloons, and baskets. Other standard accessories, such as biopsy forceps, argon plasma coagulator probes, snares, guide wires, stent guide catheters, and dilation balloons, have sufficient length and can be used with the 2-meter enteroscopes.

Given the lack of an elevator, papillary cannulation is best achieved with straight dual-lumen ERCP catheters. A long (450 cm) guide wire with a hydrophilic tip is a practical choice and allows exchange of accessories once cannulation is achieved. Exchange of accessories over the guide wire is a challenging task when using 2-meter enteroscopes, and it is not uncommon for the assistant to lose the wire. We prefer using the Autotome RX Cannulating Sphincterotome (Boston Scientific, Natick, MA, USA) before we exchange accessories. This sphincterotome allows for single-operator control where the endoscopist can hold the guide wire and avoid losing it during the long wire exchanges. The RX locking device (Boston Scientific) can also be used to lock the guide wire in place to maintain access.

The simplest and safest method for performing sphincterotomy is to initially place a biliary stent or a pancreatic stent, followed by needle knife sphincterotomy over the stent. Some endoscopists advocate performance of partial or "small" sphincterotomy followed by balloon sphincteroplasty to minimize the risk of perforation.[40]

COMPLICATIONS

The frequency of ERCP-related complications, such as pancreatitis and bleeding, are not higher in patients with altered anatomy as compared with those with normal gastrointestinal anatomy. However, because of the presence of multiple anastomoses, the perforation risk may theoretically be higher. Gerson and colleagues[41] conducted a retrospective study of DBE complications in 9 US centers. Overall, perforations occurred in 0.4% of 2478 DBE examinations. In the subset of 219 examinations performed in patients with surgically altered anatomy, perforations occurred in 3.0% (0.6% in anterograde DBE examinations). Although the DBE perforation rate was significantly elevated in patients with altered surgical anatomy, most perforations occurred during retrograde examinations in patients with surgically altered anatomy.

SUMMARY

The RYGB anatomy poses particular challenges to interventional endoscopists who intend to access the papilla. Deep enteroscopy-assisted ERCP seems to be the least invasive technique for this purpose, and is often the best initial choice. However, considerable experience is needed to optimize the success rate of reaching the biliopancreatic limb, with subsequent successful cannulation, and which approach is taken should be determined on a case-by-case basis.

REFERENCES

1. Nguyen DM, El-Serag HB. The big burden of obesity. Gastrointest Endosc 2009; 70(4):752–7.
2. Ogden CL, Yanovski SZ, Carroll MD, et al. The epidemiology of obesity. Gastroenterology 2007;132(6):2087–102.
3. Prentice AM. The emerging epidemic of obesity in developing countries. Int J Epidemiol 2006;35(1):93–9.
4. Davis MM, Slish K, Chao C, et al. National trends in bariatric surgery, 1996–2002. Arch Surg 2006;141(1):71–4 [discussion: 75].
5. Steinbrook R. Surgery for severe obesity. N Engl J Med 2004;350(11):1075–9.
6. Santry HP, Gillen DL, Lauderdale DS. Trends in bariatric surgical procedures. JAMA 2005;294(15):1909–17.
7. Trus TL, Pope GD, Finlayson SR. National trends in utilization and outcomes of bariatric surgery. Surg Endosc 2005;19(5):616–20.
8. Ward M, Prachand V. Surgical treatment of obesity. Gastrointest Endosc 2009; 70(5):985–90.
9. Shiffman ML, Sugerman HJ, Kellum JM, et al. Gallstone formation after rapid weight loss: a prospective study in patients undergoing gastric bypass surgery for treatment of morbid obesity. Am J Gastroenterol 1991;86(8):1000–5.
10. Hintze RE, Adler A, Veltzke W, et al. Endoscopic access to the papilla of Vater for endoscopic retrograde cholangiopancreatography in patients with billroth II or Roux-en-Y gastrojejunostomy. Endoscopy 1997;29(2):69–73.
11. Wright BE, Cass OW, Freeman ML. ERCP in patients with long-limb Roux-en-Y gastrojejunostomy and intact papilla. Gastrointest Endosc 2002;56(2):225–32.
12. Yamamoto H, Kita H, Sunada K, et al. Clinical outcomes of double-balloon endoscopy for the diagnosis and treatment of small-intestinal diseases. Clin Gastroenterol Hepatol 2004;2(11):1010–6.
13. Yamamoto H, Sekine Y, Sato Y, et al. Total enteroscopy with a nonsurgical steerable double-balloon method. Gastrointest Endosc 2001;53(2):216–20.
14. Sakai P, Kuga R, Safatle-Ribeiro AV, et al. Is it feasible to reach the bypassed stomach after Roux-en-Y gastric bypass for morbid obesity? The use of the double-balloon enteroscope. Endoscopy 2005;37(6):566–9.

15. Koornstra JJ. Double balloon enteroscopy for endoscopic retrograde cholangiopancreaticography after Roux-en-Y reconstruction: case series and review of the literature. Neth J Med 2008;66(7):275–9.
16. Aabakken L, Bretthauer M, Line PD. Double-balloon enteroscopy for endoscopic retrograde cholangiography in patients with a Roux-en-Y anastomosis. Endoscopy 2007;39(12):1068–71.
17. Emmett DS, Mallat DB. Double-balloon ERCP in patients who have undergone Roux-en-Y surgery: a case series. Gastrointest Endosc 2007;66(5):1038–41.
18. Moreels TG, Roth B, Vandervliet EJ, et al. The use of the double-balloon enteroscope for endoscopic retrograde cholangiopancreatography and biliary stent placement after Roux-en-Y hepaticojejunostomy. Endoscopy 2007;39(Suppl 1): E196–7.
19. Spahn TW, Grosse-Thie W, Spies P, et al. Treatment of choledocholithiasis following Roux-en-Y hepaticojejunostomy using double-balloon endoscopy. Digestion 2007;75(1):20–1.
20. Monkemuller K, Bellutti M, Neumann H, et al. Therapeutic ERCP with the double-balloon enteroscope in patients with Roux-en-Y anastomosis. Gastrointest Endosc 2008;67(6):992–6.
21. Parlak E, Cicek B, Disibeyaz S, et al. Endoscopic retrograde cholangiography by double balloon enteroscopy in patients with Roux-en-Y hepaticojejunostomy. Surg Endosc 2010;24(2):466–70.
22. Chu YC, Yang CC, Yeh YH, et al. Double-balloon enteroscopy application in biliary tract disease—its therapeutic and diagnostic functions. Gastrointest Endosc 2008;68(3):585–91.
23. Maaser C, Lenze F, Bokemeyer M, et al. Double balloon enteroscopy: a useful tool for diagnostic and therapeutic procedures in the pancreaticobiliary system. Am J Gastroenterol 2008;103(4):894–900.
24. Tsujikawa T, Saitoh Y, Andoh A, et al. Novel single-balloon enteroscopy for diagnosis and treatment of the small intestine: preliminary experiences. Endoscopy 2008;40(1):11–5.
25. Kawamura T, Yasuda K, Tanaka K, et al. Clinical evaluation of a newly developed single-balloon enteroscope. Gastrointest Endosc 2008;68(6):1112–6.
26. Ramchandani M, Reddy DN, Gupta R, et al. Diagnostic yield and therapeutic impact of single-balloon enteroscopy: series of 106 cases. J Gastroenterol Hepatol 2009;24(10):1631–8.
27. Upchurch BR, Vargo JJ. Single-balloon enteroscopy. Gastrointest Endosc Clin N Am 2009;19(3):335–47.
28. Itoi T, Ishii K, Sofuni A, et al. Single-balloon enteroscopy-assisted ERCP in patients with Billroth II gastrectomy or Roux-en-Y anastomosis (with video). Am J Gastroenterol 2010;105(1):93–9.
29. Dellon ES, Kohn GP, Morgan DR, et al. Endoscopic retrograde cholangiopancreatography with single-balloon enteroscopy is feasible in patients with a prior Roux-en-Y anastomosis. Dig Dis Sci 2009;54(8):1798–803.
30. Wang AY, Sauer BG, Behm BW, et al. Single-balloon enteroscopy effectively enables diagnostic and therapeutic retrograde cholangiography in patients with surgically altered anatomy. Gastrointest Endosc 2010;71(3):641–9.
31. Esmail S, Odstrcil EA, Mallat D, et al. A single center retrospective review of spiral enteroscopy. Gastrointest Endosc 2009;69:AB197.
32. Baron TH, Vickers SM. Surgical gastrostomy placement as access for diagnostic and therapeutic ERCP. Gastrointest Endosc 1998;48(6):640–1.

33. Brotherton AM, Judd PA. Quality of life in adult enteral tube feeding patients. J Hum Nutr Diet 2007;20(6):513–22 [quiz: 523–5].
34. Martinez J, Guerrero L, Byers P, et al. Endoscopic retrograde cholangiopancreatography and gastroduodenoscopy after Roux-en-Y gastric bypass. Surg Endosc 2006;20(10):1548–50.
35. Bannerman E, Pendlebury J, Phillips F, et al. A cross-sectional and longitudinal study of health-related quality of life after percutaneous gastrostomy. Eur J Gastroenterol Hepatol 2000;12(10):1101–9.
36. Baron TH. Double-balloon enteroscopy to facilitate retrograde PEG placement as access for therapeutic ERCP in patients with long-limb gastric bypass. Gastrointest Endosc 2006;64(6):973–4.
37. Mutignani M, Marchese M, Tringali A, et al. Laparoscopy-assisted ERCP after biliopancreatic diversion. Obes Surg 2007;17(2):251–4.
38. Roberts KE, Panait L, Duffy AJ, et al. Laparoscopic-assisted transgastric endoscopy: current indications and future implications. JSLS 2008;12(1):30–6.
39. Lopes TL, Clements RH, Wilcox CM. Laparoscopy-assisted ERCP: experience of a high-volume bariatric surgery center (with video). Gastrointest Endosc 2009;70(6):1254–9.
40. Haber GB. Double balloon endoscopy for pancreatic and biliary access in altered anatomy (with videos). Gastrointest Endosc 2007;66(Suppl 3):S47–50.
41. Gerson LB, Tokar J, Chiorean M, et al. Complications associated with double balloon enteroscopy at nine US centers. Clin Gastroenterol Hepatol 2009;7(11):1177–82, 1182,e1–3.

Current Status of Endoluminal Bariatric Procedures for Primary and Revision Indications

Marvin Ryou, MD[a,b], Michele B. Ryan, MS[c],
Christopher C. Thompson, MD[c,*]

KEYWORDS

- Bariatric endoscopy • Endoscopic revision • Obesity
- Bariatric • Primary obesity therapy • Endoscopic suturing
- Gastric volume reduction • Transoral

Endoscopic bariatric procedures are gaining traction as possible treatment modalities for obesity. A major reason for its intuitive appeal is that endoluminal obesity therapy represents a much-needed minimally invasive treatment option that is currently lacking in the management strategy of this worsening epidemic. For example, treatment of coronary artery disease spans a continuum, with cardiac stenting representing a point of intervention between medications/lifestyle changes and cardiac surgery. Similarly, for treatment of degenerative joint disease, arthroscopic surgery has an important role between medication/lifestyle changes and joint replacement surgery. By comparison, in the treatment of obesity, there is currently a glaring absence of minimally invasive options between medications/lifestyle changes, which have limited efficacy, and

---

Dr Ryou's disclosures include: Beacon Endoscopy (consultant; royalties); Covidien (consultant). Ms Ryan has nothing to disclose.
Dr Thompson's disclosures include: Bard, Bariatric Advisory Board member/research support; USGI Medical, advisory board member; Valentx, consultant; Covidien, Endoluminal Advisory Board/educational continuing medical education activity grant; Boston Scientific, consultant and medical education activity grant in the area of endoluminal operating platforms; Beacon Endoscopy (consultant, royalties).

[a] Partners Combined Program, Division of Gastroenterology, Brigham and Women's Hospital, 75 Francis Street, Boston, MA 02115, USA
[b] Gastrointestinal Unit, Massachusetts General Hospital, Boston, 55 Fruit Street, MA 02114, USA
[c] Division of Gastroenterology, Brigham and Women's Hospital, 75 Francis Street, Boston, MA 02115, USA
* Corresponding author.
E-mail address: cthompson@hms.harvard.edu

Gastrointest Endoscopy Clin N Am 21 (2011) 315–333
doi:10.1016/j.giec.2011.02.004 giendo.theclinics.com
1052-5157/11/$ – see front matter

conventional bariatric surgery, which exhibits a not insignificant morbidity and mortality profile that causes many to avoid seeking treatment.

Endoscopic bariatric procedures can potentially satisfy the need for a minimally invasive option in one or more different capacities. For example, they may be used as (1) an **early intervention** to provide weight loss or weight stabilization in early-stage obese patients who do not yet qualify for traditional bariatric surgery. Alternatively, they could be used as (2) a **bridge to surgery** to reduce operative risk for various bariatric and nonbariatric surgeries. Endoscopic bariatric procedures could also be used as (3) a primary **metabolic** treatment to address comorbid illnesses such as diabetes. Furthermore, they could be used as (4) a **primary** bariatric treatment in the traditional surgical population, with the efficacy matching the specific device risk profile. Finally, they could be used as (5) **revisional** treatment for patients requiring repair following traditional bariatric surgery (**Table 1**).[1]

This article focuses its discussion on the various endoscopic devices and procedures that pertain to the last 2 points of intervention—primary and revisional treatments. However, it is important to keep in mind that many of these devices may also be applicable to 1 or more of the other 3 categories. This aspect depends on various device-specific attributes such as safety, removability or reversibility, and effect on comorbid illness. For example, intragastric balloons may be best applied as a bridge therapy because they require removal after 6 months, whereas endoscopic suturing may have more wide-ranging applications as a primary treatment, revisional treatment, early intervention, or bridge to surgery depending on how the suturing instrument is used. Another example may include endoscopic sleeves that could be applied as both primary metabolic therapy and bridge to surgery, given that they currently require removal and achieve significant metabolic end points. This review largely focuses on the primary and revisional applications for specific devices, as the current literature is concentrated on these areas. Study results pertaining to applications in (1) early intervention, (2) bridge to surgery, and (3) primary metabolic categories are highlighted where available. Devices that are currently in human use are preferentially discussed, followed by references to devices that may see clinical use in the near future (**Table 2**).

PRIMARY TREATMENT

Intragastric Balloons

Intragastric balloons have been in use since 1982[2] as a space-occupying device to induce a sense of satiety, and they represent the most frequently placed endoscopic

Table 1
Bariatric endoscopy: different points of intervention

Procedure Category	Procedure Aim
Early intervention	Providing weight loss or stabilization in early-stage obese patients who do not yet qualify for traditional surgery
Bridge to surgery	Reducing the obesity-related operative risk for various bariatric and nonbariatric surgeries
Metabolic	Primarily addressing comorbid illness (eg, diabetes)
Primary	Endoscopic option for the traditional surgical population, with outcomes and risk profiles similar to those of current surgeries
Revision	Repairing failed bariatric surgical procedures

Data from Thompson CC. Endoscopic therapy of obesity: a new paradigm in bariatric care. Gastrointest Endosc 2010;72:505–7.

Table 2
Procedures/devices: primary, revisional, and future directions

Procedure Category	Procedures/Devices
Primary	Intragastric balloons (Allergan, Spatz-FGIA Inc, Helioscopie) RESTORe Suturing System (C.R. Bard Inc) TOGa Stapler (Satiety Inc) TERIS (Barosense) Bypass Liners (GI Dynamics, ValenTx) Incisionless Operating Platform (USGI Medical Inc)
Revision	Sclerotherapy Bard EndoCinch Suturing System (C.R. Bard Inc) Incisionless Operating Platform (USGI Medical Inc) StomaphyX (Endogastric Solutions) OverStitch (Apollo) OTSC-Clip (Ovesco AG)
Future directions	Neuromodulation Transoral anastomosis devices Devices targeting neurohormonal pathways

device to date. The BioEnterics Intragastric Balloon (BIB; Allergan, Irvine, CA, USA) has been the most extensively studied of the intragastric balloons (**Fig. 1**). The BIB is designed as a sphere to hold 400 to 800 mL of saline, and requires removal after 6 months. BIBs are currently in use worldwide, although they are not yet available in the United States; this is in part due to several complications and premature balloon deflation associated mainly with the predecessor, the Garren-Edwards Gastric Bubble (GEGB).

Studies have demonstrated weight loss in the short-term and mid-term ranges, but long-term weight loss, especially following balloon removal, has been equivocal. Genco and colleagues[3] retrospectively reviewed 2515 Italian patients and showed a 6 month excess weight loss of 33.9% ± 18.7%. However, in a randomized controlled

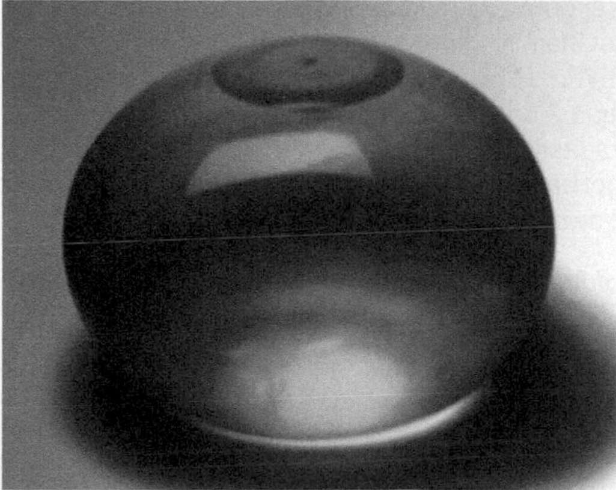

Fig. 1. BioEnterics Intragastric Balloon (BIB; Allergan, Irvine, CA). (*From* Ganesh R. Rao AD, Baladas HG, et al. The Bioenteric Intragastric Balloon (BIB) as a treatment for obesity: poor results in Asian patients. Singapore Med J 2007;48(3):227–31. This figure has been previously published in the Singapore Medical Journal [2007;48(3):227–31] and is reproduced with the kind permission of the Editor.)

trial comparing balloon treatment versus sham over a 3-month period in 43 patients (mean body mass index [BMI; calculated as the weight in kilograms divided by height in meters squared, ie, kg/m^2] of 43.3 kg/m^2), Mathus-Vliegen and Tytgat[4] found no statistical difference. Of note, after excluding 8 patients who either had not met the 3-month weight loss goal (n = 5) or did not tolerate the balloon (n = 3), the remaining balloon patients (n = 12) exhibited a mean weight loss of 21.3 kg (excess weight loss [EWL] of 17.1%) after 12 months. Following balloon removal at 12 months, these patients had still maintained weight loss of 12.6 kg (9.9%) at the end of the second, balloon-free year (with nutrition and physician counseling). In summary, this data suggests that in patients who tolerate therapy, balloon treatment could result in substantial 1-year weight loss, and the greater part of that weight loss could be maintained during a second, balloon-free year.

In another prospective study examining long-term outcomes after BIB placement, 100 consecutive morbidly obese patients were enrolled to 6 months of BIB therapy with no structured weight maintenance program following balloon removal.[5] Ninety-seven percent of patients completed a mean final follow-up of 4.8 years. After 6 months, 63% of patients had 10% or more baseline weight loss. At final follow-up, only 28% were able to maintain this. At that time, 35 patients had undergone bariatric surgery and 34 patients had no significant weight change from baseline. These findings suggested that balloon implantation may be helpful in a minority of patients for long-term weight loss without a structured weight maintenance program.

Intragastric balloons have also been used in the super-morbidly obese population as a bridge to conventional bariatric surgery. In one study, a BIB was placed in 26 high-risk superobese patients with a mean BMI of 65.3 $\pm$ 9.8 kg/m^2 and mean 4.33 $\pm$ 1.12 severe comorbidities.[6] Endoscopic placement was uneventful in all patients. However, one patient died of cardiac arrest following aspiration on the first postinsertion day. The mean weight loss was 28.5 $\pm$ 19.6 kg after the balloon was removed at 6 months. The mean reduction in comorbidity status was 4.33 to 2.23. Twenty patients underwent primary bariatric surgery the day after BIB removal, and 2 patients were rejected because of inadequate weight loss.

Intragastric balloons are designed for 6-month deployment, but recent studies suggest that repeated treatment may sustain weight loss at least to 1 year. In a prospective, nonrandomized multicenter study, patients with repeat treatment had greater weight loss than single-treatment patients at 1 year (12.0 kg vs 6.0 kg; 40.9% vs 20.8% EWL; P = .008) but this difference became dampened by the 3-year mark (less than 2 kg difference).[7]

In summary, intragastric balloons may represent a potential option for patients unwilling to undergo bariatric surgery, or as a potential bridge to bariatric surgery with an eye toward reducing perioperative risk.

Transoral Gastric Volume Reduction (TRIM Procedure) Using the Bard Suturing System

The EndoCinch device (C.R. Bard Inc, Murray Hill, NJ, USA) was the first endoscopic suturing platform used for the treatment of obesity. It was originally designed for the treatment of gastroesophageal reflux disease and then revisions of failed gastric bypass (discussed in the section on revisional treatment), and more recently for the primary treatment of obesity. The device features a hollow capsule that fits on to the endoscope tip and uses suction for tissue acquisition. A hollow needle is delivered through the acquired tissue to pass suture material back and forth. The most recent iteration of this device (the Restore Suturing System) allows for the creation of deeper, full-thickness plications and eliminates the need for device withdrawal for suture reloading as was required by its predecessor (**Fig. 2**).

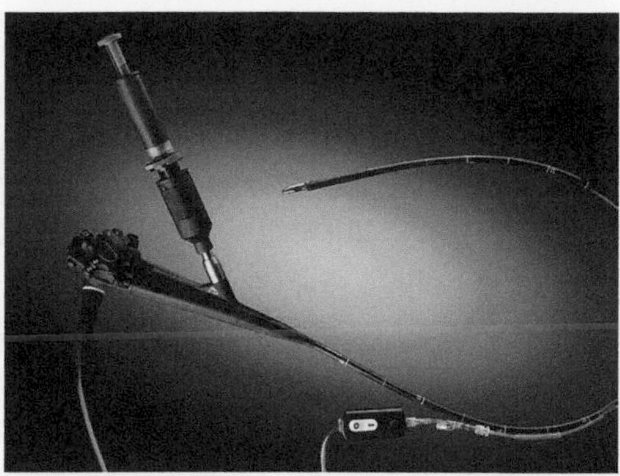

Fig. 2. Restore Suturing System (C.R. Bard Inc, Murray Hill, NJ). (*From* Brethauer SA, Chand B, Schauer PR, et al. Transoral gastric volume reduction for weight management: technique and feasibility in 18 patients. Surg Obes Relat Dis 2010;6(6):689–94; with permission.)

In 2008 Fogel and colleagues[8] published a single-center, non–United States study using the EndoCinch system to perform transoral gastric volume reduction in 64 patients with a mean BMI of 39.9 ± 5.1 kg/m^2. A running suture pattern was used to approximate a vertical gastroplasty (**Fig. 3**). The mean procedure time was 45 minutes, and no adverse events were reported. The mean %EWL at 12 months was 58.1 ± 19.9%. The mean BMI at 12 months was 30.6 ± 4.7 kg/m^2. When stratifying by original BMI groups, the patients with lowest BMI appeared to lose the most weight: BMI of 40 kg/m^2 or more had a %EWL at 12 months of 48.9 ± 10.7%. For BMI of 35 to 40 kg/m^2, the %EWL at 12 months was 56.5 ± 13.9%. For BMI less than 35 kg/m^2, the %EWL at 12 months was 85.1 ± 24.0%. These results raised the possibility of a role for transoral gastric volume reduction in early intervention of obesity.

A recent United States pilot study in 18 patients with a BMI of 30 to 56 kg/m^2 was published by Brethauer and colleagues.[9] Gastric plications were created to approximate the anterior and posterior gastric walls to achieve functional volume reduction in the gastric body and fundus (**Fig. 4**). The procedure was successfully performed in all patients. The average number of plications was 6 (range 4–8). The average procedure time was 125 ± 23 minutes. There were no serious or significant procedure-related complications. The first 10 patients were kept overnight per study protocol, and the remaining 8 were discharged on the day of the procedure. Data regarding weight loss, comorbidity improvement, and durability are currently under assessment.

In summary, the Restore Suturing Device places full-thickness gastric plications for gastric volume reduction. Early favorable results have been demonstrated in a wide range of BMI groups. Additional studies regarding durability of weight loss are forthcoming.

Transoral Gastroplasty Using the TOGa Stapling Device

The TOGa system (Satiety Inc, Palo Alto, CA, USA) uses a set of transoral endoscopically guided staplers to create a restrictive sleeve by deploying a vertical staple line along the lesser curvature (**Fig. 5**). The TOGa stapler has a flexible 18-mm diameter shaft and is introduced over a guidewire. The device accommodates a standard endoscope to provide retroflexed visualization of the procedure. A septum from the device spreads and positions the anterior and posterior gastric walls, which are then apposed using vacuum. Two successive vertical staple lines are deployed to create a partial

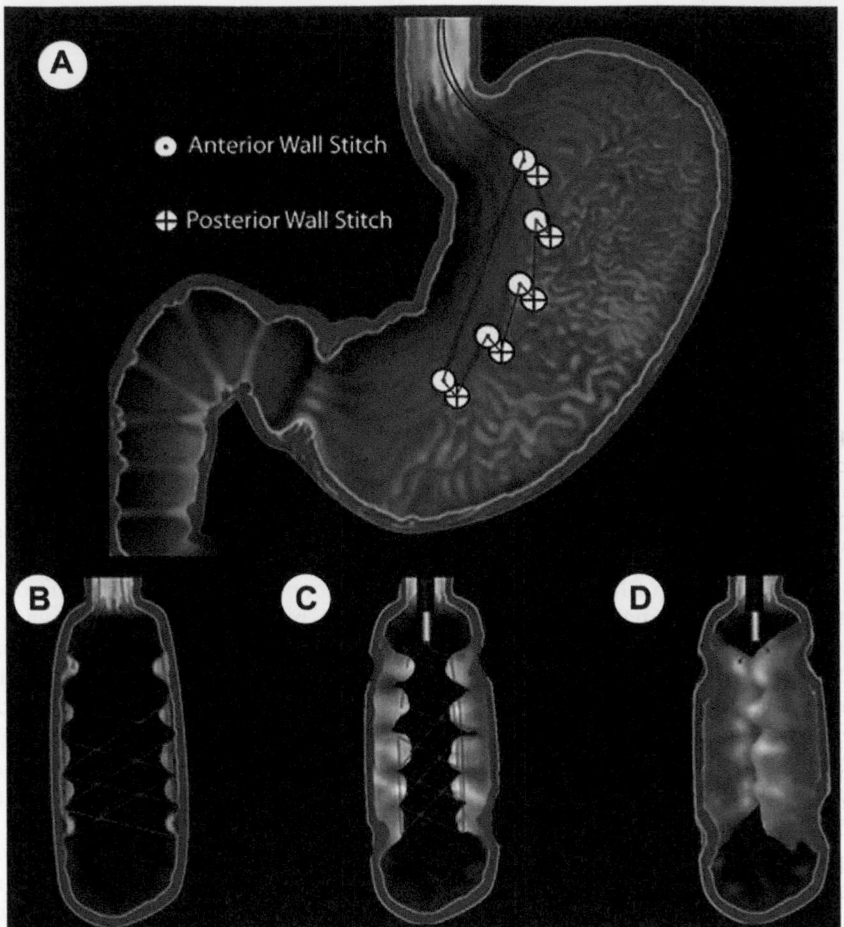

Fig. 3. Restore Suturing System. A running suture pattern was used to approximate a vertical gastroplasty. (*A*) A frontal cross-sectional view of the stomach after all stitches were placed. (*B–D*) Cross sections of the stomach as the suture is pulled tight and secured to complete the procedure. (*From* Mullady DK, Jonnalagadda S. Primary endoscopic obesity procedures. Tech Gastrointest Endosc 2010;12(3):167–76; with permission.)

sleeve approximately 8 to 9 cm in length. A "restrictor" stapler is then used to staple pleats of tissue at the inferior end of the sleeve to create a restrictive "pouch."

In a recent multicenter study enrolling 21 patients with mean BMI of 43.3 kg/m^2 (range 35–53 kg/m^2), the procedure was completed safely in all patients.[10] There were no serious adverse events. At 6-month endoscopy, all patients had full or partial stapled sleeves. However, staple line gaps were evident in 13 of the 21 patients. The average weight loss was 8 kg (16.2% EWL) at 1 month, 11.1 kg (22.6% EWL) at 3 months, and 12 kg (24.4% EWL) at 6 months.

Following technical improvement, particularly in staple line deployment, the results of a second human trial were published.[11] In 11 patients, the mean %EWL was 19% (1 month), 34% (3 months), and 46% (6 months). Average BMI decreased from 41.6 kg/m^2 preprocedure to 33.1 kg/m^2 at 6 months. Results from a multicenter, randomized, sham-controlled study are anticipated in the near future.

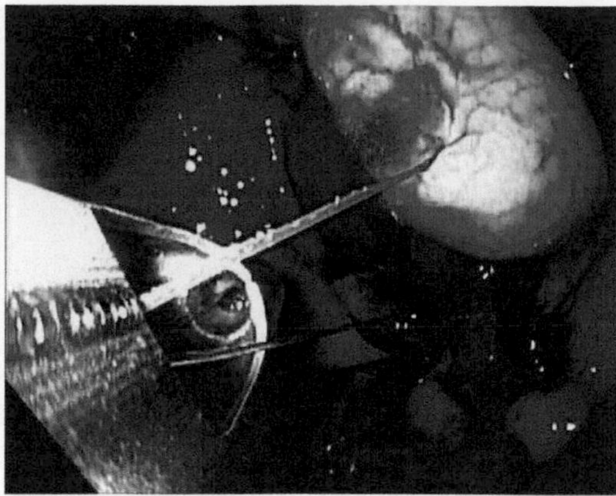

Fig. 4. Restore Suturing System. Gastric plications were created to approximate the anterior and posterior gastric walls to achieve restriction of the upper stomach. (*From* Brethauer SA, Chand B, Schauer PR, et al. Transoral gastric volume reduction for weight management: technique and feasibility in 18 patients. Surg Obes Relat Dis 2010;6(6):689–94; with permission.)

Transoral Endoscopic Restrictive Implant System

The endoscopic corollary of the gastric band, the transoral endoscopic restrictive implant (TERIS) system (Barosense Inc, Redwood City, CA, USA) is an endoscopic device designed to implant a prosthetic diaphragm in the gastric cardia via anchors to stapled plications. Although the device shares a similar location with the gastric band, the mechanism of action may in fact be rather different. The procedure involves the introduction of a stapler through an overtube to create full-thickness transmural plications in the cardia region. An anchor is then placed through a hole in the plication. This process is repeated until 5 plications with anchors are formed. The implant is then "parachuted" into place and locked to the anchors, thereby creating a gastric pouch (**Fig. 6**).

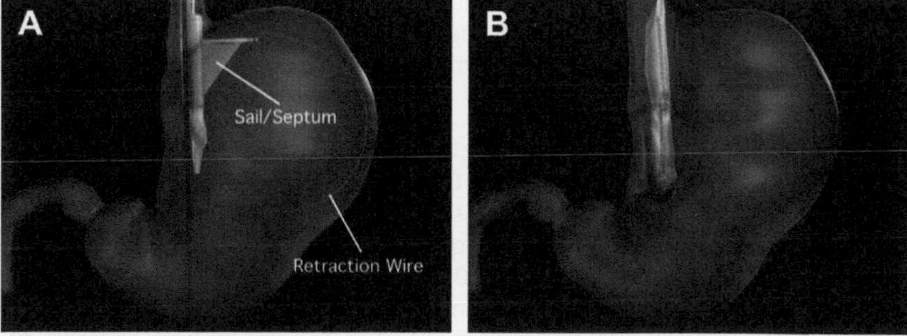

Fig. 5. TOGa System. (*A*) A depiction of the stapler in the stomach. The pediatric endoscope is positioned in the distal body and retroflexed to visualize the procedure. The stapler is advanced into the stomach, and the retraction wire and sail properly align the device to optimize opposition of the anterior and posterior gastric wall when the stapler is fired. (*B*) A second staple line is created, resulting in a 7- to 8-cm sleeve along the lesser curvature. (*From* Mullady DK, Jonnalagadda S. Primary endoscopic obesity procedures. Tech Gastrointest Endosc 2010;12(3):167–76; with permission.)

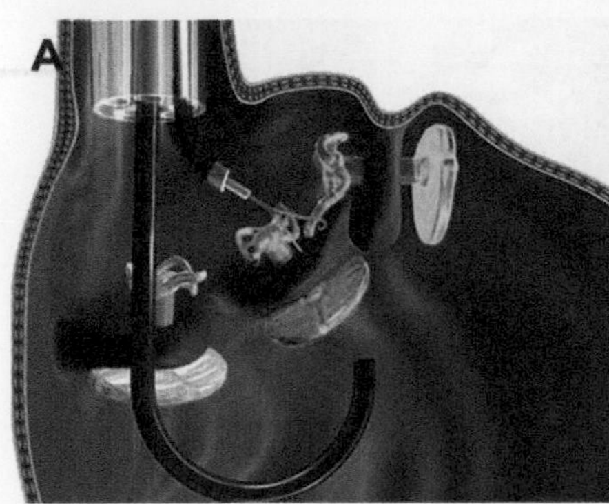

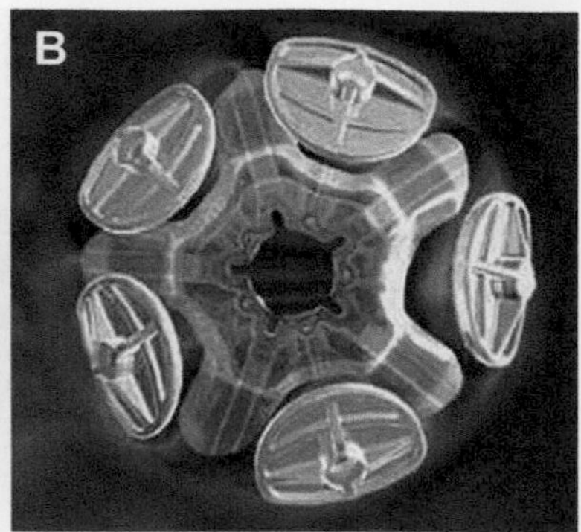

Fig. 6. TERIS System. (*A*) Placement of locking graspers on anchors. (*B*) Gastric restrictor viewed from below. (*From* Mullady DK, Jonnalagadda S. Primary endoscopic obesity procedures. Tech Gastrointest Endosc 2010;12(3):167–76; with permission.)

In a recent phase 1 pilot study involving 13 patients with median BMI of 42.1 kg/m^2, the TERIS implant was successfully deployed in 12 of the 13 patients.[12] Procedural complications occurred in 3 patients, including gastric perforation related to stapler malfunctioning in 1 patient (procedure abandoned) and pneumoperitoneum in 2 patients, treated with percutaneous needle decompression in one patient and conservative management in the other. At 3 months post procedure, the median %EWL was 28%. The median BMI had decreased from 42.1 to 37.9 kg/m^2. Further studies are under way.

Bypass Liners: the EndoBarrier and ValenTx Sleeves

Endoscopically placed bypass sleeves are generating considerable interest as a type of metabolic surgery, given the clinical observation that bypassing the proximal small bowel, as in procedures such as the Roux-en-Y gastric bypass, not only induces weight loss but also significantly improves type 2 diabetes.[13] Mounting evidence indicates that proximal intestinal diversions improve glucose homeostasis by modulation of gut hormones independent of reduced food intake and body weight.[14]

There are currently two sleeve devices in human studies. The first, the EndoBarrier gastrointestinal liner, is a bypass sleeve that is seated in the duodenum and extends into the proximal jejunum. The second, the ValenTx sleeve, implants at the gastroesophageal junction and extends into the mid jejunum, thereby bypassing the stomach as well.

EndoBarrier

The EndoBarrier gastrointestinal liner (GI Dynamics, Lexington, MA, USA) is endoscopically placed as a removable malabsorptive barrier that both blocks nutrient absorption and prevents mixing of food with biliopancreatic secretions in the duodenum (**Fig. 7**). The plastic liner is 60 cm long and extends into the proximal jejunum. It is attached to a self-expanding implant that seats in the duodenum. Recent published studies of the EndoBarrier have focused on its potential both as stand-alone primary therapy for obesity and as a bridge to bariatric surgery.

Several trials have demonstrated the potential benefit of the EndoBarrier system. A pilot study of 12 patients demonstrated successful deployment in less than 30 minutes and successful removal in 40 minutes.[15] Mean %EWL was 23.6%. Two patients required device explantation due to abdominal pain. All 4 diabetic patients who participated did not require their diabetes medications during the study duration, and all

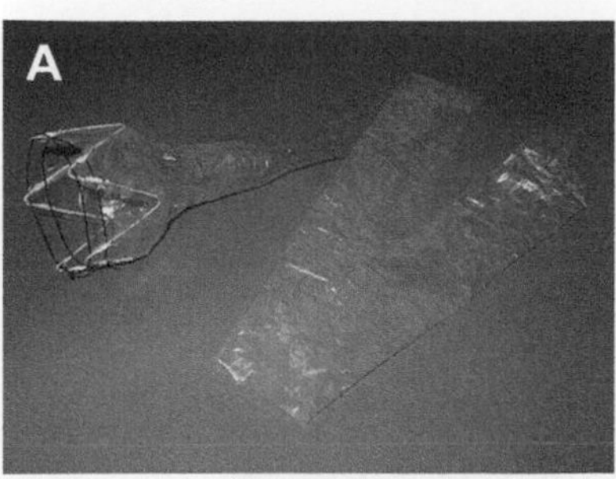

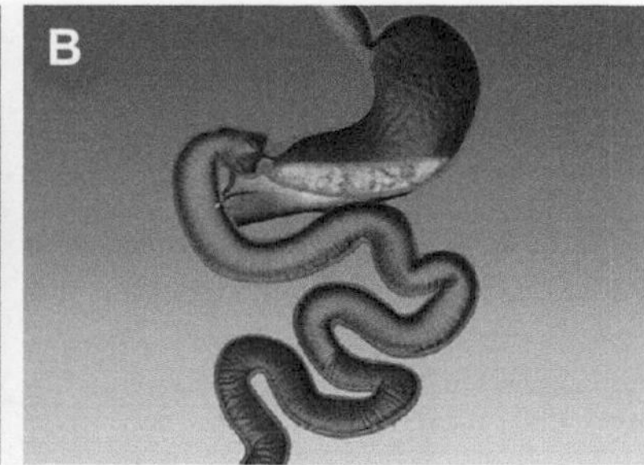

Fig. 7. (*A*) The EndoBarrier (GI Dynamics, Lexington, MA) duodenal-jejunal bypass sleeve consists of an impermeable fluoropolymer sleeve of 60 cm and a nitinol anchor with barbs. The polypropylene drawstring is necessary for removal of the device. (*B*) Illustration of the EndoBarrier gastrointestinal liner. The device is endoscopically placed in the duodenum to form a barrier between chyme and the intestinal wall, creating a duodenal-jejunal bypass effect. (*From* Mullady DK, Jonnalagadda S. Primary endoscopic obesity procedures. Tech Gastrointest Endosc 2010;12(3):167–76; with permission.)

registered significant decreases in their hemoglobin A_{1c} compared with the control group. A second, multicenter study from Chile showed significant 12-week weight loss in 24 patients treated with the EndoBarrier system compared with a diet control group (22% vs 5% EWL, respectively).[16] Of note, in this study 5 patients (20%) underwent early sleeve explantation due to bleeding (n = 3), migration (n = 1), and obstruction (n = 1). In a recent study, 10 patients underwent EndoBarrier sleeve therapy combined with a restrictor orifice (flow restrictor) for 3 months, and the mean % EWL at the conclusion of the study was 40% ± 3%.[17] The mean total weight loss was 16.7 ± 1.4 kg.

In a recent multicenter randomized clinical trial examining EndoBarrier therapy prior to conventional bariatric surgery, 41 patients were enrolled with 30 patients undergoing sleeve implantation and 11 patients serving as a diet control group.[18] Of the 30 patients randomized to sleeve therapy, 26 devices were successfully implanted and maintained for 3 months. Again, the 4 implantation failures were attributable to dislocation of the anchor (n = 1), sleeve obstruction (n = 1), sleeve migration (n = 1), and continuous epigastric pain (n = 1). Mean procedure time was 35 minutes. There were no procedure-related adverse events. Mean initial BMI was 48.9 kg/m^2 for the device group and 47.4 kg/m^2 for the control group. Mean %EWL at 3 months was 19.0% for device patients versus 6.9% for control patients ($P<.002$). Absolute change in BMI at 3 months was 5.5 kg/m^2 and 1.9 kg/m^2, respectively. Type 2 diabetes mellitus was present at baseline in 8 patients of the device group and improved in 7 patients during the study period, as evidenced by lower glucose levels, hemoglobin A_{1c}, and medication requirements.

In summary, the EndoBarrier has demonstrated significant weight loss at 12 weeks in a series of studies. It has also demonstrated considerable glycemic improvements in diabetic patients as well as potential utility as a bridge to bariatric surgery. Design modifications have been made to improve problems with bleeding, sleeve migration, and sleeve obstruction, and longer term trials are needed to answer questions about durability of response.

ValenTx sleeve

ValenTx (Valentx Inc, Carpinteria, CA, USA) is a device that consists of a 120-cm sleeve secured at the gastric cardia (**Fig. 8**).[19] The device ultimately extends into

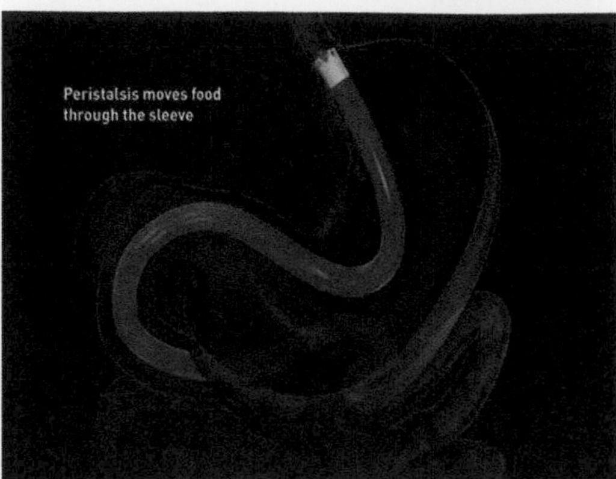

Fig. 8. ValenTx sleeve (Valentx Inc, Carpinteria, CA). (*Courtesy of* ValenTx; with permission.)

the mid-jejunum. The sleeve is impermeable and does not allow for proximal small bowel nutrient absorption. Metabolic effects occur when undigested material is presented to the mid small bowel. The device is currently implanted as a hybrid procedure, with endoscopic suturing under laparoscopic visualization. A critical part of this procedure is careful site selection and positioning of the internal cuff.

Early results from a pilot study were presented in abstract form in 2010. The study enrolled 22 patients, with 17 patients able to maintain the device for the full 12 weeks. The primary reason for early explantation was dysphagia. Mean %EWL at 8 weeks was 40.5%, and 39.9% at 12 weeks. Seven patients with preoperative diabetes mellitus all had normal blood glucose levels throughout the trial and none required antihyperglycemia medications. Hemoglobin A_{1c} levels improved for all enrolled diabetic patients.

Incisionless Operating Platform/POSE Procedure

The Incisionless Operating Platform (IOP; USGI Medical Inc, San Clemente, CA, USA) is a multifunctional endoscopic platform that has been applied to primary obesity therapy in a procedure called Primary Obesity Surgery, Endoluminal, or POSE (**Fig. 9**). The IOP uses a specialized overtube with 4 channels—one for the endoscope itself and 3 for endoscopic instruments. One endoscopic instrument is a combined grasper with a curved hollow needle for tissue anchor deployment. The grasper has large jaws (2.5 cm in length) allowing for robust tissue acquisition and creation of full-thickness tissue plications. Plications are placed within the gastric body and fundus to reduce gastric volume.

A United States registry of POSE patients is under way, and results have not yet been reported. Presentation of early clinical results is anticipated in 2011.

REVISIONAL TREATMENT

Although Roux-en-Y gastric bypass is considered one of the most effective weight loss procedures, up to 20% of bypass patients will fail to meet success criteria (defined as >50% EWL within 1 year of surgery)[20] and up to 20% of bypass patients will experience significant weight regain (>15% from nadir).[21] The causes for failed Roux-en-Y gastric bypass are likely multifactorial, but mechanical causes such as dilation of the gastrojejunal anastomosis and/or gastric pouch are thought to contribute through loss of restriction. Recent studies have demonstrated that larger size of the gastric pouch[22] and larger diameter of the gastrojejunal stoma[23,24] correlate

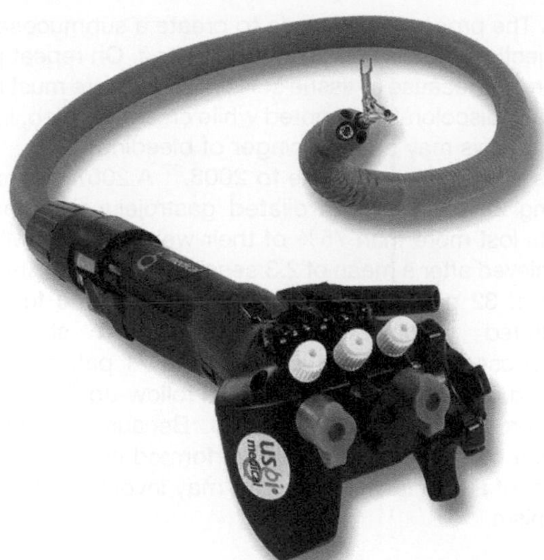

Fig. 9. Incisionless Operating Platform (IOP) (USGI Medical Inc, San Clemente, CA). (*Courtesy of* USGI Medical Inc; with permission.)

with increased weight gain. Surgical revision for weight regain following gastric bypass has a reported complication rate of 15% to 50% using standard approaches.[25,26] Endoluminal revision of dilated gastrojejunal stomas and dilated gastric pouches theoretically has a lower risk profile and may provide a solution to some patients struggling with this problem.

Sclerotherapy

Sclerotherapy is a revisional therapy based on the injection of sclerosant in peristomal tissue (**Fig. 10**). Using an endoscopic injection needle, sodium morrhuate is injected around the gastrojejunal anastomosis. This procedure is repeated at 8- to 12-week intervals and often requires a total of 2 to 3 sessions to achieve the desired outlet size of less than 12 mm. Approximately 2 mL per injection for a total of up to 20 mL

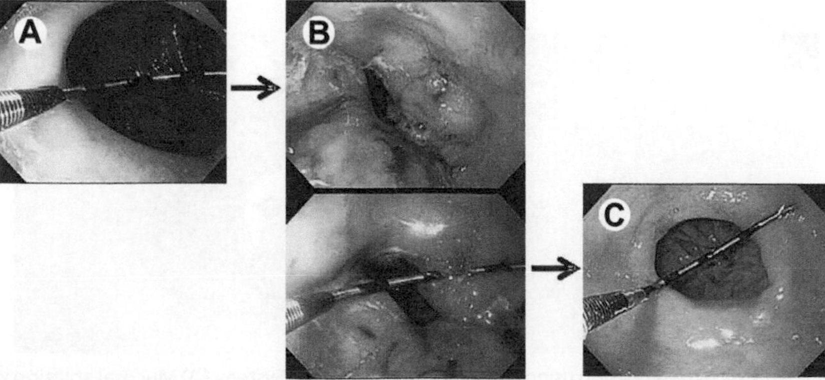

Fig. 10. Gastrojejunostomy anastomosis (*A*) before and (*B*) immediately after sclerotherapy injections, and (*C*) 3 months after procedure. (*From* Woods KE, Abu Dayyeh BK, Thompson CC. Endoscopic post-bypass revisions. Tech Gastrointest Endosc 2010;12(3):160–6; with permission.)

per session is best. The proper technique is to create a submucosal bleb in the area and to avoid overinjection, as this may lead to bleeding. On repeat procedures blebs may be difficult to create because of tissue sclerosis, and care must be taken. Of note, if dark maroon or black discoloration is noted while creating a bleb, injection should be halted immediately, as this may be a harbinger of bleeding.

Published studies of sclerotherapy date to 2003.[27] A 2007 gastrointestinal endoscopy study involving 28 patients with dilated gastrojejunal stomas demonstrated that 64% of patients lost more than 75% of their weight regain following nadir. This weight loss was achieved after a mean of 2.3 sessions.[28] A 2007 study retrospectively examined a cohort of 32 patients with 1-year follow-up and found that 91.6% of patients demonstrated weight loss and/or weight stabilization following sclerotherapy.[29] A subsequent 2008 study involving 71 patients showed that 72% of patients maintained or lost weight at 12-month follow-up.[30]

Sclerotherapy is procedurally straightforward. Because it uses standard endoscopic accessories, it could theoretically be performed in most endoscopy centers. Its exact mechanism of action is unknown and may involve more than restoration of a restrictive mechanism.

Bard EndoCinch Suturing System

In addition to primary obesity therapy, the Bard EndoCinch Suturing System (C.R. Bard Inc, Murray Hill, NJ, USA) can be used for revision of dilated gastrojejunal anastomoses. Again, the device features a hollow capsule that fits onto the endoscope tip and uses suction for tissue acquisition. A hollow needle is delivered through the acquired tissue to pass suture material back and forth. For revision of a dilated gastrojejunostomy, the device is used to place several interrupted stitches around a gastrojejunal outlet, after the stomal rim has undergone mucosal ablation with argon plasma coagulation (**Fig. 11**).

Use of the Bard EndoCinch Suturing System for revision of dilated gastrojejunal anastomosis was initially reported in 2006.[31] In this pilot study, 8 patients with a mean BMI of 40.5 kg/m^2, an average stoma diameter of 25 mm, and significant post-bypass weight regain (average 24 kg from nadir) were included. The average post-reduction anastomosis diameter was 10 mm. Six patients experienced a mean weight loss of 10 kg at 4 months. Repeat procedures were performed on 3 subjects. Of those repeat reduction patients, 2 subjects showed a total weight

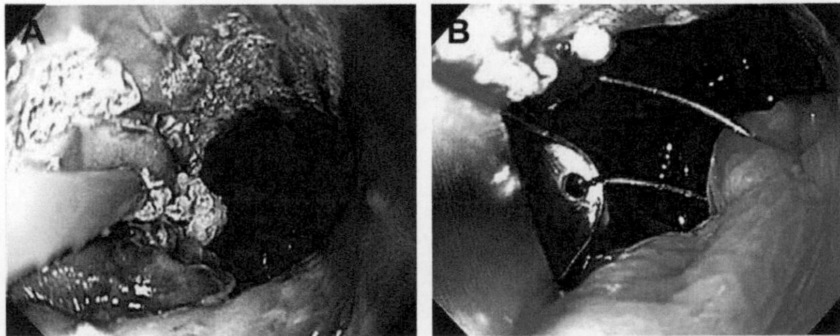

Fig. 11. Gastric bypass revision using the EndoCinch Suturing System. (*A*) Mucosal ablation with argon plasma coagulation. (*B*) Placement of sutures. (*From* Thompson CC, Slattery J, Bundga ME, et al. Peroral endoscopic reduction of dilated gastrojejunal anastomosis after Roux-en-Y gastric bypass: a possible new option for patients with weight regain. Surg Endosc 2006;20(11):1744–8; with kind permission from Springer Science+Business Media.)

loss of 19 kg and 20 kg, respectively, at 5 months. Out of the 11 total reduction procedures, no significant complications occurred. Average post-reduction BMI was 37.7 kg/m^2 and %EWL was 23.4%.

In a randomized, double-blinded, sham-controlled United States multicenter trial (the RESTORe trial), 77 patients with mean BMI of 47.6 kg/m^2 were randomized to either transoral sutured revision of a dilated gastrojejunal stoma (>20 mm) or sham procedure.[32] Technical success was achieved in 89% of cases (reduction of stoma to <10 mm). There were no deaths or perforations. Patients were followed for 6 months. Two patients randomized to the suturing group could not undergo the procedure but were kept blinded. Within this as-treated analysis, mean weight loss for the sutured group was 4.7% $\pm$ 5.7% versus 1.9% $\pm$ 5.2% (P = .041). Mean weight loss using a last observation carried forward intent-to-treat analysis was 4.2% $\pm$ 5.4% and 1.9% $\pm$ 5.2% (P = .066). Weight loss or weight stabilization was achieved in 96% of the intervention group. The intervention group also demonstrated a reduction in both systolic and diastolic blood pressure as well as a trend toward improvement in metabolic indices.

It is noteworthy that the EndoCinch Suturing System has also been used for treatment of gastrogastric fistulae, another cause of weight regain following Roux-en-Y gastric bypass. In a study of 95 patients who underwent gastrogastric fistulae closure either with endoscopic suturing (n = 71; 75%) or endoscopic clipping (n = 24; 25%), complete initial fistula closure was achieved in 9 0 patients (95%) with reopening in 59 (65%) after an average of 177 $\pm$ 202 days. Patients with fistulae less than 10 mm in diameter had the best long-term results.[33]

Incisionless Operating Platform/ROSE Procedure

The IOP can be used for revision (ROSE procedure) of dilated gastric pouches and dilated gastrojejunal stomas. The system is the same that already described for POSE; however, the procedure is different from a technical standpoint. Plications are placed around a dilated stoma or within a dilated gastric pouch instead of within the gastric body and fundus (**Fig. 12**).

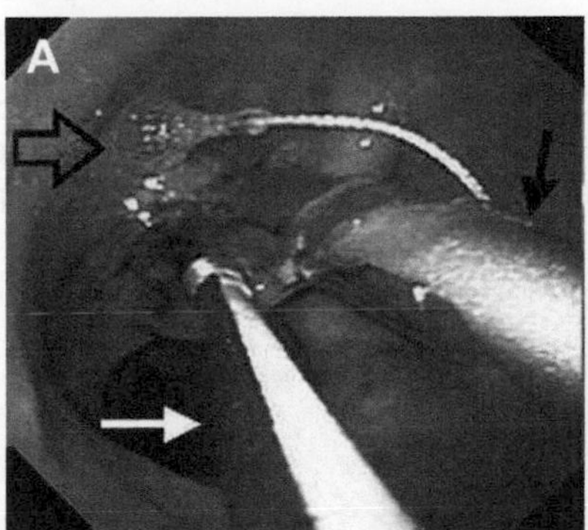

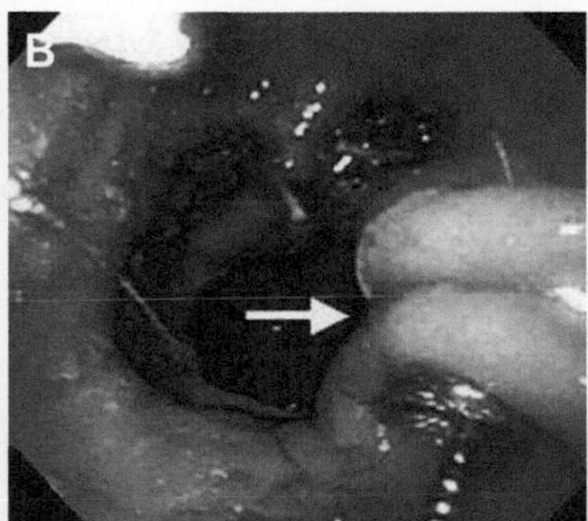

Fig. 12. ROSE procedure. (*A*) After tissue is grasped at rim of the gastrojejunal anastomosis with a corkscrew-like tissue grasper (*white arrow*), the g-Prox (USGI Medical) is closed on tented tissue (*black arrow*) and the first anchor is deployed (*open arrow*). (*B*) after the g-Prox is released from the tissue, the second anchor is deployed, creating a tissue plication (*arrow*). (*From* Mullady DK, Lautz DB, Thompson CC. Treatment of weight regain after gastric bypass surgery when using a new endoscopic platform: initial experience and early outcomes (with video). Gastrointest Endosc 2009;70(3):440–4; with permission.)

Early prospective United States studies publishing the use of the IOP for post-bypass pouch and stoma reduction were first mentioned in 2009.[34,35] Both of these studies demonstrated technical feasibility and minimal procedural complications. Mullady and colleagues[35] reported technical success in 85% of the cases (17/20), with a mean weight loss in successful cases of 8.8 kg at 3 months, while Ryou and colleagues[34] reported technical success in 100% of patients (5/5) using a second-generation device, with a mean weight loss in successful cases of 7.8 kg at 3 months.

More recently, in a prospective United States multicenter registry study, 116 patients were followed over 1 year following endoluminal revision using the IOP.[36] These patients had regained significant weight more than 2 years following Roux-en-Y gastric bypass after losing at least 50% of the excess body weight following Roux-en-Y. This patient cohort had also been screened for stomal and/or pouch dilation. Anchors were successfully placed in 112 (97%) patients with an intraoperative reduction of stomal diameter and pouch length of 50% and 44%, respectively. The average procedure time was 87 minutes. No significant complications occurred. At 6 months after the procedure, an average of 32% of weight regain that had occurred after Roux-en-Y gastric bypass had been lost. The average %EWL was 18%. Twelve-month endoscopies confirmed the retention of anchors and durable plications.

StomaphyX

The StomaphyX device (EndoGastric Solutions Inc, Redmond, WA, USA) is a single-use endoluminal device for ligasure-based creation of plications in the gastric pouch (**Fig. 13**). The device uses suction for tissue acquisition and delivers polypropylene H-fasteners to secure full-thickness plications. These plications are created in a circumferential manner in the gastric pouch, thereby reducing pouch volume.

In a recent study of 39 patients with average BMI of 39.8 kg/m^2, average %EWL at 1 month was 10.6% (n = 34); 13.1% at 3 months (n = 15); 17.0% at 6 months (n = 14); and 19.5% at 12 months (n = 6).[37] Minor complications included transient sore throat in 87% of patients and transient epigastric pain in 76.9% of patients. In another study with 64 patients, the mean weight loss was 7.6 kg at a mean follow-up of 5.8 months.[38]

OverStitch Endoscopic Suturing System

The OverStitch (Apollo Endosurgery, Austin, TX, USA) is in part an evolution of the original Eagle Claw suturing device (**Fig. 14**). The OverStitch mounts onto the tip of a double-channel therapeutic gastroscope and uses a curved needle to deploy

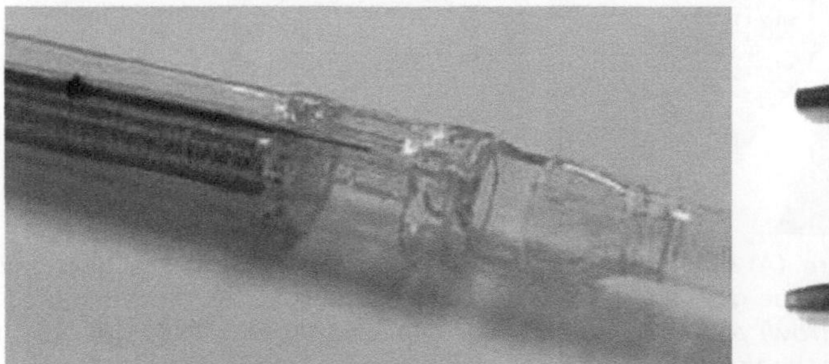
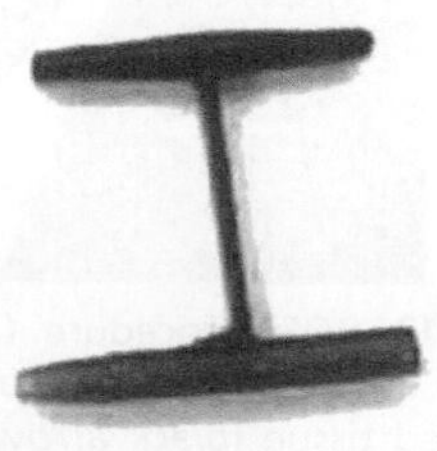

Fig. 13. StomaphyX delivery system and H-shaped polypropylene pledget. (EndoGastric Solutions, Inc, Redmond, WA). (*From* Woods KE, Abu Dayyeh BK, Thompson CC. Endoscopic post-bypass revisions. Tech Gastrointest Endosc 2010;12(3):160–6; with permission.)

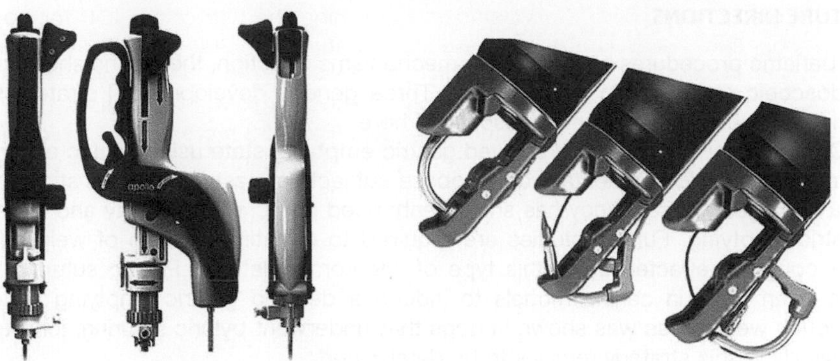

Fig. 14. OverStitch (Apollo Endosurgery, Austin, TX). (*Courtesy of* Apollo Endosurgery; with permission.)

full-thickness sutures under direct visualization. Single-handed operation of suture deployment allows for the endoscopist to control the depth of suture placement while also maintaining visibility of the operative site. The device can deploy a running stitch as well as interrupted sutures, and can also be reloaded without scope removal.

The OverStitch has demonstrated clinical versatility in its early human feasibility studies. It has been used in oversewing of chronic marginal ulcers and closure of various fistulae. In addition, the OverStitch has been used for revision of dilated gastrojejunostomy in 9 patients, which was recently submitted in abstract form. Preliminary results are promising, and longer term studies are under way.

OTSC(R)-Clip

An endoscopic over-the-scope clip (OTSC(R); Ovesco AG, Tubingen, Germany) has also been used to reduce the size of the gastrojejunal anastomosis (**Fig. 15**). In a recent study of 94 patients following gastric bypass with a starting mean BMI of 32.8 $\pm$ 1.9, the mean 3-month BMI was 29.7 $\pm$ 1.8 kg/m^2, and the mean 1-year BMI was 27.47 $\pm$ 3.8 kg/m^2.[39] Best clinical results were obtained by narrowing the gastrojejunostomy by placing 2 clips at opposite sites, thereby reducing the outlet by more than 80%.

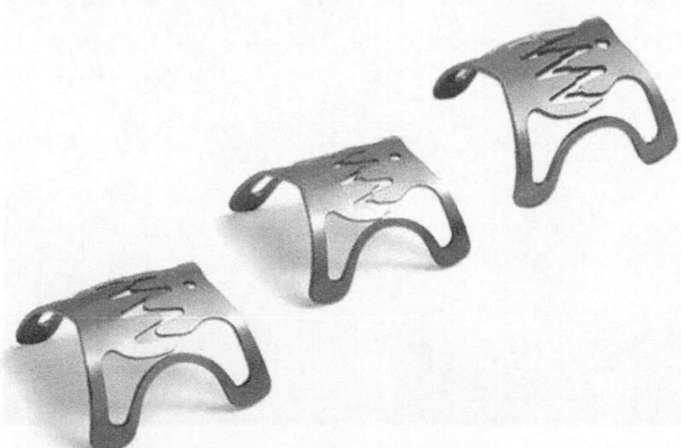

Fig. 15. Endoscopic over-the-scope clip (OTSC(R); Ovesco AG, Tubingen, Germany). (*From* Heylen AM, Jacobs A, Lybeer M, et al. The OTSC(R)-Clip in revisional endoscopy against weight gain after bariatric gastric bypass surgery. Epub ahead of print 2010 Sep. With kind permission from Springer Science+Business Media.)

FUTURE DIRECTIONS

As bariatric procedures have complex mechanisms of action, there is no shortage of endoscopic strategies in development. Three general developmental strategies in various stages of evaluation are discussed here.

One strategy is to induce a delayed gastric emptying state using gastric electrical stimulation.[40,41] Experimental work in obese subjects of gastric electrical stimulation at a tachygastrial frequency has shown enhanced postprandial satiety and delayed gastric emptying. Further studies are required to quantify the type of weight loss that could be effected using this type of "neuromodulation." Pyloric suturing has also been used in canine models to induce a delayed gastric emptying state.[42] Although weight loss was shown in dogs that underwent pyloric suturing, long-term feasibility of this strategy remains to be determined.

A second developmental strategy is to endoscopically recreate the most effective bariatric postsurgical anatomies, such as Roux-en-Y gastric bypass anatomy. An example is smart self-assembling magnets for endoscopy (SAMSEN) used for transoral creation of gastrojejunal anastomoses (**Fig. 16**).[43] Following endoscopic delivery, these magnets self-assemble into predetermined configurations (eg, square or hexagon). When reciprocal macromagnets occupy 2 different hollow organs (eg, stomach and jejunum), they align and mate to create an anchoring window that can be cut through for an instant anastomosis. Compression anastomosis allows for the creation of a robust, large-caliber fistula after several days, and the magnets are then sloughed off. The implications for weight loss and for metabolic end points with such approaches are obvious.

Finally, endoscopic strategies specifically targeting the neurohormonal pathways of obesity may represent the most effective treatment options of the future, but will certainly require the most development. Potential targets include ghrelin response to fasting or postprandial ghrelin inhibition and/or stimulation of appetite suppressant, such as peptide YY or glucagon-like peptide 1. Enhanced understanding of physiologic effects of key component(s) of various bariatric surgeries and newer endoluminal therapies will undoubtedly allow more refined design of treatment options in the future.[44]

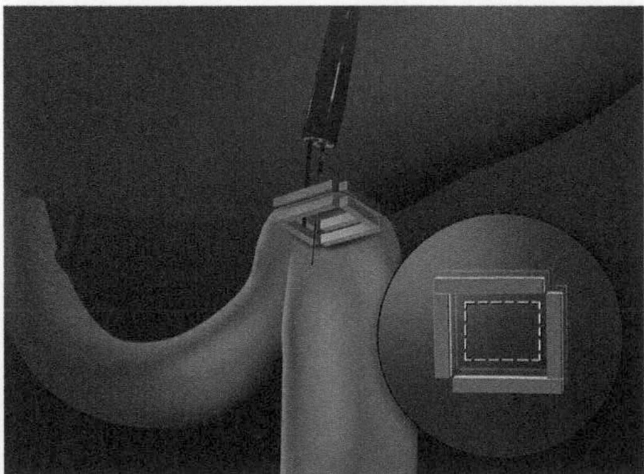

Fig. 16. Smart self-assembling magnets for endoscopy (SAMSEN) used for transoral creation of gastrojejunal anastomoses. (*From* Ryou M, Cantillon-Murphy P, Azagury D, et al. Smart Self-Assembling Magnets for Endoscopy (SAMSEN) for transoral endoscopic creation of immediate gastrojejunostomy (with video). Gastrointest Endosc 2011;73(2):353–9; with permission.)

SUMMARY

Endoluminal bariatric procedures meet a glaring need for a minimally invasive option in the treatment of obesity. Given the increasing scope of endoluminal bariatrics, the gastroenterologist stands to play an important role in the treatment of obesity. Numerous devices and technologies are currently being developed, modified, and evaluated in early human studies. These procedures can potentially be offered as early interventions in premorbidly obese patients; as bridges to surgery to reduce operative risk; as primary metabolic therapies; as primary weight-loss procedures; or as revisional treatments of failed bariatric surgery. It is important for gastroenterologists to become more involved with the care of bariatric patients now, so that they better understand the disease and are fully equipped to assume more responsibility in the management of this condition in the future.

REFERENCES

1. Thompson CC. Endoscopic therapy of obesity: a new paradigm in bariatric care. Gastrointest Endosc 2010;72:505–7.
2. Nieben OG, Harboe H. Intragastric balloon as an artificial bezoar for treatment of obesity. Lancet 1982;1:198–9.
3. Genco A, Bruni T, Doldi SB, et al. Bioenterics intragastric balloon: the Italian experience with 2515 patients. Obes Surg 2005;15:1161–4.
4. Mathus-Vliegen EM, Tytgat GN. Intragastric balloon for treatment-resistant obesity: safety, tolerance, and efficacy of 1-year balloon treatment followed by a 1-year balloon-free follow-up. Gastrointest Endosc 2005;61:19–27.
5. Dastis NS, Francois E, Deviere J, et al. Intragastric balloon for weight loss: results in 100 individuals followed for at least 2.5 years. Endoscopy 2009;41: 575–80.
6. Spyropoulos C, Katsakoulis E, Mead N, et al. Intragastric balloon for high-risk super-obese patients: a prospective analysis of efficacy. Surg Obes Relat Dis 2007;3:78–83.
7. Dumonceau JM, Francois E, Hittelet A, et al. Single vs repeated treatment with the intragastric balloon: a 5-year weight loss study. Obes Surg 2010;20:692–7.
8. Fogel R, de Fogel J, Bonilla Y, et al. Clinical experience of transoral suturing for an endoluminal vertical gastroplasty: 1-year follow-up in 64 patients. Gastrointest Endosc 2008;68:51–8.
9. Bretahuer SA, Chand B, Schauer PR, et al. Transoral gastric volume reduction for weight management: technique and feasibility in 18 patients. Surg Obes Relat Dis 2010;6:689–94.
10. Deviere J, Ojeda Valdes G, Cuevas Herrera L, et al. Safety, feasibility and weight loss after transoral gastroplasty: first human multicenter study. Surg Endosc 2008;22:589–98.
11. Moreno C, Closset J, Dugardeyn S, et al. Transoral gastroplasty is safe, feasible, and induces significant weight loss in morbidly obese patients: results of the second human pilot study. Endoscopy 2008;40:406–13.
12. de Jong K, Mathus-Vliegen EM, Veldhuyzen EA, et al. Short-term safety and efficacy of the Trans-oral Endoscopic Restrictive Implant System for the treatment of obesity. Gastrointest Endosc 2010;72:497–504.
13. Rubino F, Forigone A, Cummings DE, et al. The mechanism of diabetes control after gastrointestinal bypass surgery reveals a role of the proximal small intestine in the pathophysiology of type 2 diabetes. Ann Surg 2006;244:741–9.

14. Rubino F, Schauer PR, Kaplan LM, et al. Metabolic surgery to treat type 2 diabetes: clinical outcomes and mechanisms of action. Annu Rev Med 2010;61:393–411.
15. Rodriguez-Grunert L, Galvao Neto MP, Alamo M, et al. First human experience with endoscopically delivered and retrieved duodenal-jejunal bypass sleeve. Surg Obes Relat Dis 2008;4:55–9.
16. Tarnoff M, Rodriguez L, Escalona A, et al. Open label, prospective, randomized controlled trial of an endoscopic duodenal-jejunal bypass sleeve versus low calorie diet for pre-operative weight loss in bariatric surgery. Surg Endosc 2009;23:650–6.
17. Escalona A, Yanez R, Pimentel F, et al. Initial human experience with restrictive duodenal-jejunal bypass liner for treatment of morbid obesity. Surg Obes Relat Dis 2010;6:126–31.
18. Schouten R, Rijs CS, Bouvy ND, et al. A multicenter, randomized efficacy study of the EndoBarrier Gastrointestinal Liner for presurgical weight loss prior to bariatric surgery. Ann Surg 2010;251:236–43.
19. Sandler BJ, Swain CP, Rumbaut R, et al. First human experience with endoluminal, endoscopic gastric bypass [abstract]. Surg Endosc 2010;24:S226–7.
20. Brolin RE. Bariatric surgery and long-term control of morbid obesity. JAMA 2002; 288:2793–6.
21. McCormick JT, Papsavas PK, Caushaj PF, et al. Laparoscopic revision of failed open bariatric procedures. Surg Endosc 2003;17:413–5.
22. Roberts K, Duffy A, Kaufman J, et al. Size matters: gastric pouch size correlates with weight loss after laparoscopic Roux-en-Y gastric bypass. Surg Endosc 2007; 21:1397–402.
23. Mali J Jr, Fernandes FA, Valezi AC, et al. Influence of the actual diameter of the gastric pouch outlet in weight loss after silicon ring Roux-en-Y gastric bypass: an endoscopic study. Obes Surg 2010;20:1231–5.
24. Dayyeh BK, Lautz DB, Thompson CC. Gastrojejunal stoma diameter predicts weight regain after Roux-en-Y gastric bypass. Clin Gastroenterol Hepatol 2011; 9:228–33.
25. Coakley BA, Deveney CW, Spight DH, et al. Revisional bariatric surgery for failed restrictive procedures. Surg Obes Relat Dis 2008;4:581–6.
26. Gagner M, Gentileschi P, de Csepel J, et al. Laparoscopic reoperative bariatric surgery: experience from 27 consecutive patients. Obes Surg 2002;12:254–60.
27. Spaulding L. Treatment of dilated gastrojejunostomy with sclerotherapy. Obes Surg 2003;13:254–7.
28. Catalano MF, Rudic G, Anderson AJ, et al. Weight gain after bariatric surgery as a result of a large gastric stoma: endotherapy with sodium morrhuate may prevent the need for surgical revision. Gastrointest Endosc 2007;66:240–5.
29. Spaulding L, Osler T, Patlak J. Long-term results of sclerotherapy for dilated gastrojejunostomy after gastric bypass. Surg Obes Relat Dis 2007;3:623–6.
30. Loewen M, Barba C. Endoscopic sclerotherapy for dilated gastrojejunostomy of failed gastric bypass. Surg Obes Relat Dis 2008;4:539–42.
31. Thompson CC, Slattery J, Bundga ME, et al. Peroral endoscopic reduction of dilated gastrojejunal anastomosis after Roux-en-Y gastric bypass: a possible new option for patients with weight regain. Surg Endosc 2006;20(11):1744–8.
32. Thompson CC, Roslin MS, Bipan C, et al. RESTORe: randomized evaluation of endoscopic suturing transorally for anastomotic outlet reduction: a double-blind, sham-controlled multicenter study for treatment of inadequate weight loss or weight regain following Roux-en-Y gastric bypass. Gastroenterology 2010;138(5 Suppl 1):S-388.

33. Fernandez-Esparrach G, Lautz DB, Thompson CC. Endoscopic repair of gastrogastric fistula after Roux-en-Y gastric bypass: a less-invasive approach. Surg Obes Relat Dis 2010;6:282–8.
34. Ryou MK, Mullady DK, Lautz DB, et al. Pilot study evaluating technical feasibility and early outcomes of second-generation endosurgical platform for treatment of weight regain after gastric bypass surgery. Surg Obes Relat Dis 2009;5(4):450–4.
35. Mullady DK, Lautz DB, Thompson CC. Treatment of weight regain after gastric bypass surgery when using a new endoscopic platform: initial experience and early outcomes (with video). Gastrointest Endosc 2009;70(3):440–4.
36. Horgan S, Jacobsen G, Weiss GD, et al. Incisionless revision of post-Roux-en-Y bypass stomal and pouch dilation: multicenter registry results. Surg Obes Relat Dis 2010;6:290–5.
37. Mikami D, Needleman B, Narula V, et al. Natural orifice surgery: initial US experience utilizing the StomaphyX device to reduce gastric pouches after Roux-en-Y gastric bypass. Surg Endosc 2010;24:223–8.
38. Letiman IM, Virk CS, Avgerinos DV, et al. Early results of trans-oral endoscopic placation and revision of the gastric pouch and stoma following Roux-en-Y gastric bypass surgery. JSLS 2010;14:217–20.
39. Heylen AM, Jacobs A, Lybeer M, et al. The OTSC(R)-Clip in revisional endoscopy against weight regain after bariatric gastric bypass surgery. Obes Surg 2010. [Epub ahead of print].
40. Liu J, Hou X, Song G, et al. Gastric electrical stimulation using endoscopically placed mucosal electrodes reduces food intake in humans. Am J Gastroenterol 2006;101:798–803.
41. Wang J, Song J, Hou X, et al. Effects of cutaneous gastric electrical stimulation on gastric emptying and postprandial satiety and fullness in lean and obese subjects. J Clin Gastroenterol 2010;44:335–9.
42. Vegesna A, Korimilli A, Besetty R, et al. Endoscopic pyloric suturing to facilitate weight loss: a canine model. Gastrointest Endosc 2010;72:427–31.
43. Ryou M, Cantillon-Murphy P, Azagury D, et al. Smart Self-Assembling Magnets for Endoscopy (SAMSEN) for transoral endoscopic creation of immediate gastrojejunostomy (with video). Gastrointest Endosc 2011;73(2):353–9.
44. Stylopoulos N, Aguirre V. Mechanisms of bariatric surgery and implications for the development of endoluminal therapies for obesity. Gastrointest Endosc 2009;70: 1167–75.

Regulatory and Reimbursement Issues Regarding Endoscopic Bariatric Procedures

Steven D. Schwaitzberg, MD

KEYWORDS

• Obesity • Endoscopic therapy • Regulatory issue
• Reimbursement

From a patient's perspective, there is no doubt that a hierarchy of preferential treatment strategies exists. Undoubtedly, most patients would prefer a medical solution (their own compliance notwithstanding) for their problem, with invasive surgical solutions regarded as a last resort. Endoscopic solutions fall in between these 2 and are associated with unique benefits and challenges that will require special attention to not only patients' selection but also reimbursement. The exciting innovations that have placed new therapeutic options at our doorsteps will never come to pass into the clinical mainstream if the regulatory and payer environment is not successfully navigated. Confrontational strategies between innovators who are trying to bring new therapies forward and the regulatory bodies charged with patient safety or the payers responsible for reimbursement are potentially doomed. It is important to establish effective dialog among key stakeholders to determine the appropriate benchmarks, regulatory approval, and reimbursement.

CROSSING THE CHASM FROM INNOVATION TO MAINSTREAM

When the spark of an idea is fanned into the flame of an invention, there is a long pathway before the blaze of the mainstream therapy can be realized. Chief among the initial tasks is the adequate intellectual protection of the new idea if specific novel devices are required. This task takes the form of a patent and requires specialized legal advice if protection for the inventors, both domestically and internationally, is to be achieved. This intellectual property problem is less important in terms of financial considerations if the new procedure designed does not require novel instrumentation;

Harvard Medical School, Department of Surgery, Cambridge Health Alliance, 1493 Cambridge Street, Cambridge, MA 02139, USA
E-mail address: sschwaitzberg@challiance.org

Gastrointest Endoscopy Clin N Am 21 (2011) 335–342
doi:10.1016/j.giec.2011.02.009 giendo.theclinics.com

however, regulatory and reimbursement considerations may still prove formidable. Novel devices require prototype development and preclinical testing, which will require some level of capital investment even if a company is yet to be formed. Visionaries and early adopters will go to work in the laboratory with early device iterations to determine clinical feasibility. There are unique characteristics to these innovators that complicate whether their interest/approval has relevance to mainstream clinical introduction. For instance, the early adopters tend to be tinkerers who will to work through obstacles, whereas the mainstream tends to want solutions nicely packaged for immediate deployment. The potential for mainstream acceptance (ie, does it work, can I afford it, and can the average practitioner perform the procedure?) is a core consideration around the acquisition of the additional financial backing required to fully develop a novel device concept into a therapeutic product.

The Food and Drug Administration (FDA) has created 3 classes of devices defining increasing regulatory oversight: I, II, and III.[1] The requirements for gastroenterology are contained in the Code of Federal Regulations (CFR) Title 21—Part 876. *Gastroenterology-Urology Devices.*[2] Most class I devices can be marketed without extensive regulatory filing (eg, endoscopic bite block). Class II devices usually are marketed through the 510(k) process in which substantial equivalence to a preexisting (predicate) device is established and are *cleared* (not approved) by the FDA for marketing (eg, endoscopic ingestible capsule wireless gastrointestinal imaging system). Class III devices require premarket approval (PMA). The Enteryx injectable polymer for treatment of gastroesophageal reflux was *approved* by the PMA process in 2003. (It was subsequently recalled voluntarily by the manufacturer.)

Most unproven therapeutic interventions or those with insufficient data are classified in this last category. Human subject data are usually required after the review of adequate preclinical testing has been submitted. Performing human subject research to support a PMA with unapproved devices will generally require the issuance of an investigational device exemption (IDE) by the FDA that is applied for usually by a company but occasionally by individual investigators. A successful clinical trial will bring the innovators and the FDA together in what is referred to as a panel meeting. Members of the FDA and panel members selected as experts in the field review the PMA submission and the human subject data obtained under the IDE. They review safety data and determine whether the company's proposed claim is supported by the data on the PMA. The FDA is required to review data derived from "adequate and well-controlled tests to establish both safety and effectiveness before a new drug (or device) can be approved (marketed) for sale" (CFR Title 21, Sections 355, 360c). FDA *approval* is only for the proposed claims and results in specific labeling for the use of the device. Their specific strategies are used to obtain optimal labeling language. Attempts to secure very broad labeling may be rejected by the FDA in favor of more conscripted wording. Excessively narrow labeling prevents using the device in reasonable related situations. Once the FDA has either cleared or approved the device, manufacturers are given the green light to market and sell devices with specific labeling indications. Even if a significant cohort of clinicians use a device for off-label indications, the manufacturer may not *market* that device for such purposes. Contrary to what most people believe, the FDA itself is not funded by the federal government to test drugs or devices and relies on the data submitted by the manufacturers to support claims of safety and efficacy. FDA clearance or approval is necessary but not sufficient for reimbursement.

Once the device is approved or cleared for marketing, there is a clear split in terms of reimbursement. If the device represents a new procedure, then the reimbursement pathway is centered around the procedural reimbursement. If the device is simply a tool that enables the performance of an already approved procedure, then reimbursement is far more straightforward. The manufacturer simply attempts to convince hospitals, operating rooms, or endoscopy suites to purchase their device. This latter scenario has the benefit of avoiding the maze associated with procedural reimbursement. In some countries, the patients purchase these devices directly if the endoscopist or surgeon determines these as essential to the procedure. Procedural reimbursement is far more complex, time consuming, and expensive to achieve. It literally can be conceived of as a maze that device manufacturers must navigate to get reimbursed for their devices.[3]

Endoscopic procedures for the treatment of morbid obesity can be divided into 3 categories. Some procedures will require a specific and unique device that was created to do the procedure. In many ways, the device is the procedure. In this instance, a procedural code will need to be created because of the innovation. This new code could be relatively specific such that no other device could use the same designation or could be more general such that the predicate device is the first in a class of new procedures that could conceivably be covered by the same current procedural terminology (CPT) codes that are developed and maintained by the American Medical Association (AMA). Alternatively, new procedures could be developed as distinct services that require no special equipment to be innovated or even used outside the established labeling. For instance, there are distinct CPT codes for laparoscopic Roux-en-Y gastric bypass (43644 and 43645); yet, it is generally performed with instrumentation devised for other gastrointestinal procedures.

Unless the patient pays for a procedure out of his or her pocket, a CPT code is necessary for reimbursement. It is tempting for innovators (manufacturers, proceduralists, and hospitals) to try to use existing CPT codes as the centerpiece of their reimbursement strategy once any existing FDA requirements have been met. In the case of new operations/endoscopic procedures without novel or off-label use instrumentation, the FDA is not a factor because this body does not regulate procedures per se except through the regulation and controls placed on devices used in procedures. One way to achieve reimbursement for these emerging procedures is to use the catchall 99 unlisted procedure code for the relevant anatomic group, which will result in an individual review by the payer and more often than not a denial of payment, requiring an appeal to achieve reimbursement. As a global strategy for reimbursement of an endoscopic procedure for the treatment of morbid obesity, this is a highly labor intensive approach and is unlikely to result in mainstream adoption of any given procedure. Another approach will be to use an existing code for a distinct service listed in the current volume. The wisdom, risk, or outright danger of this approach will depend on the matchup between the proposed procedure and the description of the existing coded procedure. For example, EndoGastric Solutions (Redwood City, CA, USA) has manufactured a device created for the Esophyx procedure for the endolumenal treatment of gastroesophageal reflux. This device is marketed as a transoral incisionless fundoplication. Could a strategy be used that makes a case that the anatomic result is indistinguishable from a laparoscopic Nissen fundoplication as a rationale for using the 43280 code for Nissen reimbursement, or should the 43499 Unlisted procedure, esophagus code be used? The former is consistently well reimbursed, and casual readers of the procedure note may not notice the discrepancy initially. This issue is the same as that of applying 43243 (Upper gastrointestinal endoscopy; with injection sclerosis of esophageal and/or gastric varices) when injecting Botox for achalasia. The technical aspects of the 2 procedures are identical; however, the descriptor of the code assignment for 43243 refers to the treatment of varices, which is not a component of the treatment of achalasia. Thus, it is not recommended to use this code despite the reasonable similarities. This impact will require careful consideration for surgeons and endoscopists who seek reimbursement for novel procedures even in the absence of dedicated devices. Another pathway to the development of the procedure will be to use an existing device in a fashion not precisely covered in the labeling. In this instance, the roles of the FDA and institutional review board (IRB) are subject to some degree of interpretation. Using a device in an off-label fashion to solve a particular clinical problem of a single patient is an *innovation* not subject to review of the IRB unless the prospective proposed use is so far afield that the risks and benefits are truly unknown. On the other hand, collecting data on these devices will require human subject *research* to be performed, subject to the auspices of the IRB, and the classification of such a device must be described accurately noting that the cleared/approved device is being used in an off-label fashion. Creating a restrictive procedure by using an endolumenal suturing device and plicating the stomach may or may not prove to be effective as therapy for weight loss and will create unique challenges for reimbursement that at a minimum it will require some form of data collection (ie, research) to establish a new CPT code.

If a new CPT code is needed for a novel procedure, an application to the CPT editorial panel is required. The AMA Board of Trustees appoints 17 members from clinical experts, the insurance industry, Centers for Medicare and Medicaid Services (CMS), and the American Hospital Association. The CPT editorial panel is supported by the CPT advisory committee. These physicians are nominated by the medical specialty societies that are represented in the AMA House of Delegates and those in the AMA Health Care Professionals Advisory Committee. Requests for new codes or revisions are sent to the CPT staff of the AMA, and if meritorious, they will be sent to the CPT advisory committee where the details and data are reviewed and a determination is made if a recommendation to the CPT editorial panel for a code revision or a new code is needed.

Three categories of codes are available. Category I codes describe a distinct procedure or service with a 5-digit code and a descriptor. This category is generally what is necessary (but not always sufficient) for reimbursement. Once a category I code is assigned, it is sent to the AMA/Specialty RVS Update Committee (RUC) for valuation where relative value units (RVUs) are assigned. Category II codes are 4-digit and fifth–alpha character tracking codes used for performance measurement. Category III codes were developed in 2001, are assigned by the CPT editorial panel to emerging technologies or procedures as temporary or T codes, and are also used for tracking purposes to assess use before considering a category I assignment. The CPT editorial panel will consider limited data such as a specialty society recommendation, a clinical trial, or relevant literature as sufficient documentation to take the issue into consideration. RVUs are not assigned by the RUC and, as is discussed later, present a conundrum of technology diffusion that is directly relevant for the emerging endoscopic treatment of morbid obesity.

Clinician innovators and/or device manufacturers who have successfully scaled the twin peaks of the FDA and the CPT editorial panel may still find themselves on financial life support in need of a cash infusion to sustain the business model or appease hospital administrators who are unwilling to allow clinicians to perform unreimbursed procedures. Thus, despite prototyping, device iteration, preclinical and clinical evaluations, and the mountains of paperwork produced to overcome those hurdles, reimbursement for innovative therapies is considered individually by each payer. In the past, some small companies attempting to bring a new therapy forward have financially bled to death from nonpayment, despite FDA clearance/approval and a category I CPT code. Medicare designates part A payments to hospitals and part B payments to physicians. Although it is improving, separate groups determine if a part A or part B payment is to be made and may come to differing conclusions. Payments by Medicare are considered on a state-by-state basis by private carriers (who often aggregate several states) who are contracted with CMS to administrate payments and benefits but who can function independently unless a national coverage determination is deliberately sought, which means that, for example, a procedure might be reimbursed in Nebraska (Noridian Administrative Services) but not in Massachusetts (National Heritage Insurance Corporation) because different contractors administrate these states. Each commercial insurer reviews a proposed new procedure independently also. Thus, there are no unified approaches to reimbursement by commercial payers particularly in the absence of consistent reimbursement by CMS. Each company will have to be approached individually, although prioritizing whom to contact is usually based on local market share.

The history of devices used in the endoscopic treatment of gastroesophageal reflux highlights potential pitfalls that may beset the endoscopic treatment of morbid obesity. The worst case scenario is the development of specific policies denying coverage for procedures despite category I CPT codes. For instance, Aetna's *Clinical Policy Bulletin #213: Gastroesophageal Reflux Disease (GERD): Treatment Devices*[4] relegates most transesophageal treatment of gastroesophageal reflux as investigational and without coverage. Similar policies exist for statewide Blue Cross Blue Shield organizations citing these therapies as investigational regardless of FDA approval/clearance or simply as not medically necessary. The result is financial nonviability if the manufacturer is a small company as seen with Curon Medical or NDO Surgical.[5]

THE PAYMENT CONUNDRUM

Endolumenal therapies potentially have several basic appeals compared with conventional open or laparoscopic interventions for the primary treatment of morbid obesity. These treatments are clearly less invasive, less painful, less costly, and associated with shorter inpatient stays. In addition, there are likely less frequent and less severe complications. If so, these endoscopic therapies should be appealing to payers; however, the experience with the therapies for gastroesophageal reflux suggests a difficult road ahead for reimbursement. The problem is that these therapies are possibly less effective and less permanent. Thus, the conundrum is that the payer community is uncertain about what to do with a therapy that is potentially less expensive but possibly less effective and/or may need to be repeated or advanced to a more standard approach. The idea that an endoscopic therapy could be used as a bridge to conventional therapy has been proffered. Understandably, the last thing that the insurers want is another layer of therapy or diagnostics inserted in the treatment regimen of a given disease unless some aspect of care is reduced or eliminated. For example, this potential additional financial explains some of the caution displayed by the payers to reimburse computed tomography (CT) coronary angiography. Despite the noninvasive appeal of this technique compared with cardiac catheterization, it is unclear whether sufficient numbers of the invasive procedure can be avoided. The problem for the payers is that FDA and CPT category I assignment is rarely based on sufficient numbers in the approval data that the assessment of the financial impact of adoption can be made. Although new therapies hold promise, the lack of longitudinal data or, in some cases, a clear mechanism of action (despite empirical results) leaves critics free to recommend payment rejection despite that the cost of conventional operative care can be many fold more expensive or dangerous. The cost of generating these large numbers of patients over several years without reimbursement can be prohibitive. Initial patient trials for a new treatment rarely focus on the financial aspects of care. Many device-related trials reflect iterative development of the instrument and/or procedure. The NDO plicator used in GERD therapy was in the midst of being explored for greater efficacy of 2 plications to improve outcome when the veritable plug was pulled. The battle of reimbursement (and thus often corporate survival) seems to be a Catch-22, which, in part, is the conundrum of the T code. Although it is clear that AMA denies any assumption that procedures with T codes should not be paid, the practice is clear. In general, reimbursement for category III codes is spotty at best and is considered by some to be a straight shot to noncoverage. Why is this? There is some historical basis for the reticence of the payers to pay for the first blush of innovation. The sad reality is that the first salvo of innovation aimed at a new procedure or problem was often unsuccessful or just a first step in an iterative process. This reality has created problems for the successors in the same or related lines of work.

HISTORICAL CONSIDERATIONS

The history of a particular innovation can have a profound impact on subsequent reimbursement. Consider the first series of intragastric balloons placed for the treatment of obesity reported by Nieben and Harboe[6] in 1982. The potential simplicity of this technique was appealing; however, during that decade, other series were reported with air-filled balloons, noting limited efficacy and significant complications. The technique was ultimately abandoned.[7–12] Current iterations of the intragastric balloon will have to overcome this legacy. For instance, Medicare currently has a national noncoverage policy for the intragastric balloon in the treatment of morbid obesity. Even successes in the 2005 clinical trial require interpretation. First of all, the balloon was replaced every 3 months (what is the payment model for this?), and second, approximately 25% of the patients dropped out of the trial.[13] These facts, in the context of previous failure, will dampen the enthusiasm for reimbursement, perhaps creating an even higher bar to overcome in the form of greater numbers of patients or longer term outcome before approval for payment.

ENDOSCOPIC THERAPY AS REVISIONAL SURGERY

Patients who require revisional surgery after laparoscopic surgery, particularly Roux-en-Y gastric bypass, face procedures with significant morbidity and mortality.[14,15] A variety of endoscopic techniques have been used to treat weight gain after Roux-en-Y gastric bypass.[16–20] The appeal of endoscopic techniques in this situation is unmistakable. Unfortunately, unlike stricture dilation, in which clear CPT codes exist, there are no current codes for endoscopic treatment of an excessively dilated gastrojejunostomy or closure of a gastrogastric fistula. Because all these endoscopic procedures require advanced endoscopic instrumentation, there is commonly a significant expense. For instance, the cost of the StomaphyX procedure, which is used to plicate a dilated gastrojejunostomy, is in the $9000 to $10,000 range,[21] which is a significant out-of-pocket expense if not covered by insurance. The prospects for coverage at present are highly variable and will often be disappointing for individuals seeking these therapies. In June 2010, Horizon Blue Cross Blue Shield of New Jersey issued the updated policy concerning bariatric surgery entitled Surgery for Morbid Obesity.[22] Endolumenal revision techniques are considered investigational and thus not covered. A similar policy exists for United Healthcare[23] and Medicare. As noted previously, attempts to secure coverage using similar codes are a short-term strategy that could lead to retroactive denial of payment or potentially more recursive actions. The conundrum here is that unlike primary surgical treatment of obesity for which standard therapies exist, the currently approved approaches are unappealing for patients and surgeons in many instances because of the increased risk and difficultly. In the absence of the large numbers of patients that commodity procedures generate, the pathway to approval seems unclear, time consuming, and excessively expensive—all of which burden the patients, physicians, and hospitals. The prospect that large numbers of endoscopic therapies will be paid for out of pocket by patients seems unlikely. Certainly, this strategy failed when applied to antireflux therapy. One could speculate that obesity treatment may fare better. The cosmetic surgery market is estimated at $10 billion.[24] The existence of approved therapies (albeit more invasive) that are covered will likely result in a small self-pay market at best. The possible exception to this is revisional surgery for dilated gastrojejunostomy or gastrogastric fistula, for which the conventional option is potentially morbid. There is a need to develop a shared risk approach to these types of problems that will allow patients to be treated (if they desire), providers to be paid (at least partially), and payers to acquire data and mitigate financial risk for unsuccessful approaches.

SUMMARY

With millions of potential patients worldwide in need of effective treatment of morbid obesity, the appeal of endoscopic approaches to this problem and to the problem of revisional surgery is indisputable. Most of these approaches require a high level of technology application and technical skill, which may limit diffusion on a global scale except to wealthier patients. The payment hurdles for insured patients in the United States are considerable because of the conservative nature of the payer community. This reticence is because of a history of past failures in this and closely related arenas. In addition, the novelty of the idea of bridging therapy in the morbid obesity paradigm, which has traditionally focused on destination surgical therapies, has not yet been accepted. Finally, the idea of a less morbid approach that might require repeated applications has yet to be put to the test of economic and clinical outcome analyses that will be required for acceptance by the payers regardless of what model of health care payment (ie, fee for service, capitation, or accountable care) emerges in the future. Despite these obstacles, a pathway for innovation in health care that will allow promising technology to move forward for transparent analysis is needed for the society, ultimately rejecting those that are ineffective and promoting those that improve health—some of which are at risk for being lost in the payment conundrum.

REFERENCES

1. Available at: http://www.fda.gov/MedicalDevices/DeviceRegulationandGuidance/Overview/default.htm. Accessed September 15, 2010.
2. Available at: http://www.accessdata.fda.gov/scripts/cdrh/cfdocs/cfcfr/CFRSearch.cfm?fr=876.1075. Accessed September 15, 2010.
3. Schwaitzberg SD. Reimbursement for new technologies: the GERD maze is not patient-friendly. Medscape J Med 2008;10:14.
4. Available at: http://www.aetna.com/cpb/medical/data/200_299/0213.html. Accessed September 10, 2010.
5. Available at: http://www.bcbsms.com/com/bcbsms/apps/PolicySearch/views/ViewPolicy.php?&blank&action=viewPolicy&noprint=yes&path=%2Fpolicy%2Femed%2FTransesophageal+Endoscopic+Therapies+for+GRD.html&keywords=%3C!123-321!%3E&source=emed&page=id=169&me=index.php. Accessed September 2, 2010.

6. Nieben OG, Harboe H. Intragastric balloon as an artificial bezoar for treatment of obesity. Lancet 1982;1:198.
7. Benjamin SB. Small bowel obstruction and the Garren-Edwards gastric bubble: an iatrogenic bezoar. Gastrointest Endosc 1988;34:463.
8. Boyle TM, Agus SG, Bauer JJ. Small intestinal obstruction secondary to obturation by a Garren gastric bubble. Am J Gastroenterol 1987;82:51.
9. Kirby DF, Mills PR, Kellum JM, et al. Incomplete small bowel obstruction by the Garren-Edwards gastric bubble necessitating surgical intervention. Am J Gastroenterol 1987;82:251.
10. Meshkinpour H, Hsu D, Farivar S. Effect of gastric bubble as a weight reduction device: a controlled, crossover study. Gastroenterology 1988;95:589.
11. Miller-Catchpole R. Diagnostic and therapeutic technology assessment. Garren gastric bubble. JAMA 1986;256:3282.
12. Ulicny KS Jr, Goldberg SJ, Harper WJ, et al. Surgical complications of the Garren-Edwards gastric bubble. Surg Gynecol Obstet 1988;166:535.
13. Mathus-Vliegen EM, Tytgat GN. Intragastric balloon for treatment-resistant obesity: safety, tolerance, and efficacy of 1-year balloon treatment followed by a 1-year balloon-free follow-up. Gastrointest Endosc 2005;61:19.
14. Brolin RE, Cody RP. Weight loss outcome of revisional bariatric operations varies according to the primary procedure. Ann Surg 2008;248:227.
15. Gagner M, Gentileschi P, de Csepel J, et al. Laparoscopic reoperative bariatric surgery: experience from 27 consecutive patients. Obes Surg 2002;12:254.
16. Herron DM, Birkett DH, Thompson CC, et al. Gastric bypass pouch and stoma reduction using a transoral endoscopic anchor placement system: a feasibility study. Surg Endosc 2008;22:1093.
17. Himpens J, Cremer M, Cadiere GB, et al. Use of a new endoluminal device in the transoral endoscopic surgical procedure for the treatment of weight regain after Roux-en-Y gastric bypass. Emerging Technology Oral. Las Vegas (NV): SAGES; 2007 [abstract: #15].
18. Spaulding L. Treatment of dilated gastrojejunostomy with sclerotherapy. Obes Surg 2003;13:254.
19. Spaulding L, Osler T, Patlak J. Long-term results of sclerotherapy for dilated gastrojejunostomy after gastric bypass. Surg Obes Relat Dis 2007;3:623.
20. Thompson CC, Slattery J, Bundga ME, et al. Peroral endoscopic reduction of dilated gastrojejunal anastomosis after Roux-en-Y gastric bypass: a possible new option for patients with weight regain. Surg Endosc 2006;20:1744.
21. Mann, D. Understanding Transoral ROSE and StomaphyX Weight Loss Surgery Revision Procedures. Available at: http://www.yourbariatricsurgeryguide.com/bariatric-surgery-revision/. Accessed September 10, 2010.
22. Horizon BCBSNJ Uniform Medical Policy Surgery Policy 022. Available at: http://myprogramforlife.com/blogs/horizon-bcbs-new-jersey-changes-weight-loss-surgery-policy. Accessed August 2, 2010.
23. United Healthcare Medical Policy: bariatric Surgery no. 2011T0362K. Available at: https://www.unitedhealthcareonline.com/ccmcontent/ProviderII/UHC/en-US/Assets/ProviderStaticFiles/ProviderStaticFilesPdf/Tools%20and%20Resources/Policies%20and%20Protocols/Medical%20Policies/Medical%20Policies/Bariatric_Surgery.pdf. Accessed August 2, 2010.
24. Smith A. Cosmetic surgery market stands firm. CNNMoney.com Feb 20, 2008. Available at: http://money.cnn.com/2008/02/07/news/companies/vanity/index.htm. Accessed August 13, 2010.

Index

Note: Page numbers of article titles are in **boldface** type.

Gastrointest Endoscopy Clin N Am 21 (2011) 343–350
doi:10.1016/S1052-5157(11)00024-9 giendo.theclinics.com
1052-5157/11/$ – see front matter

P

Q

R

S

T

Moving?

Make sure your subscription moves with you!

To notify us of your new address, find your **Clinics Account Number** (located on your mailing label above your name), and contact customer service at:

Email: journalscustomerservice-usa@elsevier.com

800-654-2452 **(subscribers in the U.S. & Canada)**
314-447-8871 **(subscribers outside of the U.S. & Canada)**

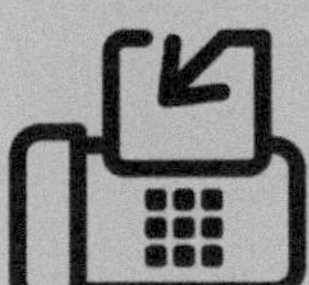

Fax number: 314-447-8029

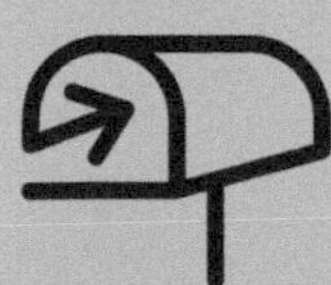

Elsevier Health Sciences Division
Subscription Customer Service
3251 Riverport Lane
Maryland Heights, MO 63043

*To ensure uninterrupted delivery of your subscription, please notify us at least 4 weeks in advance of move.

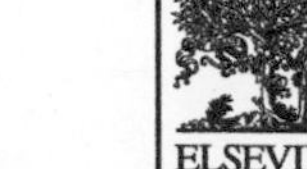

Printed and bound by CPI Group (UK) Ltd, Croydon, CR0 4YY

Printed and bound by CPI Group (UK) Ltd, Croydon, CR0 4YY

03/10/2024

01040459-0015